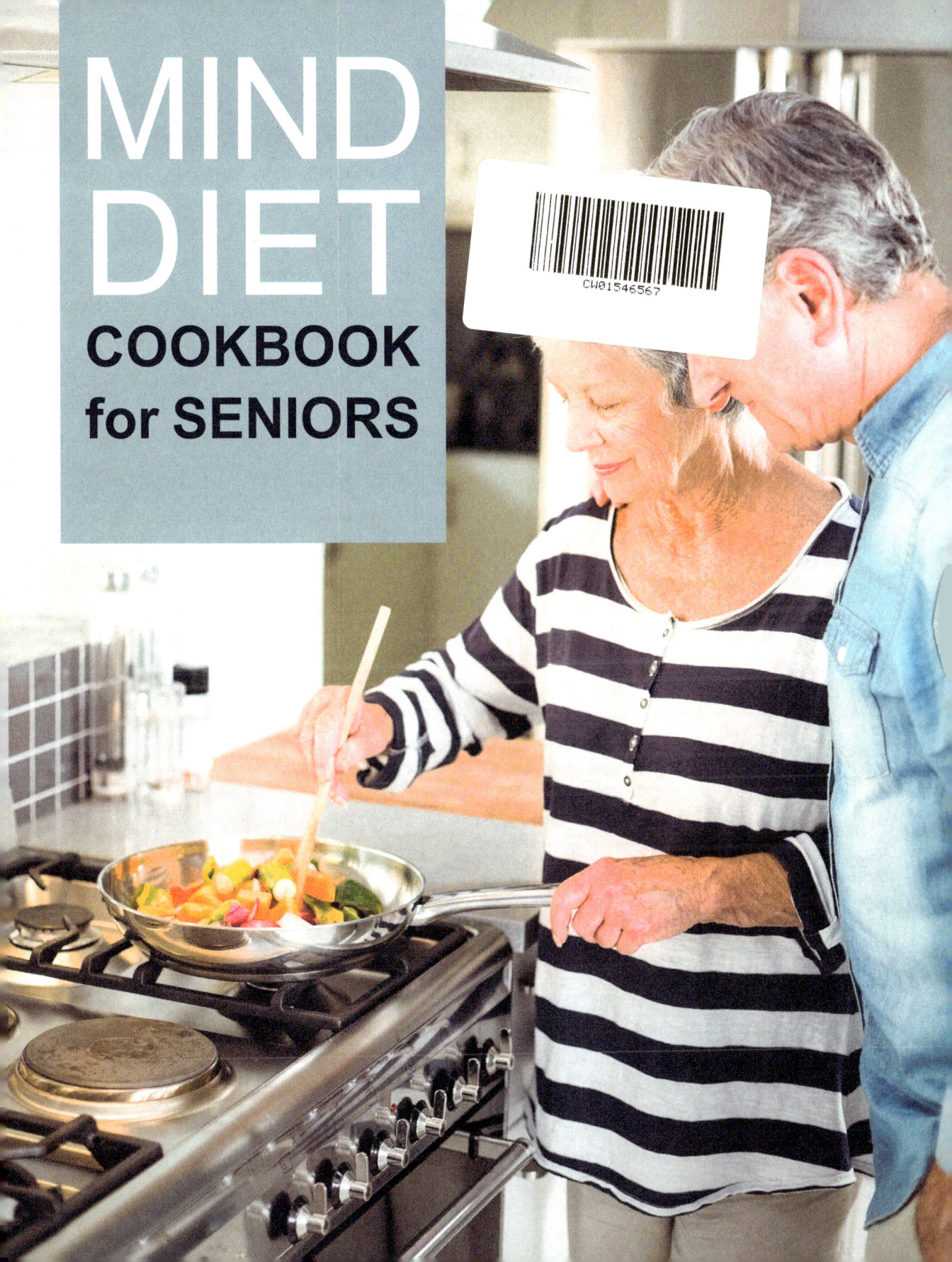

TEXT COPYRIGHT © Samuel Hartwell

All rights reserved. No part of this guide may be reproduced in any form without permission in writing from the publisher except in the case of brief quotations embodied in critical articles or reviews.

LEGAL & DISCLAIMER

The information contained in this book and its contents is not designed to replace or take the place of any form of medical or professional advice; and is not meant to replace the need for independent medical, financial, legal, or other professional advice or services, as may be required. The content and information in this book has been provided for educational and entertainment purposes only.

The content and information contained in this book has been compiled from sources deemed reliable, and it is accurate to the best of the Author's knowledge, information, and belief. However, the Author cannot guarantee its accuracy and validity and cannot be held liable for any errors and/or omissions. Further, changes are periodically made to this book as and when needed. Where appropriate and/or necessary, you must consult a professional (including but not limited to your doctor, attorney, financial advisor, or such other professional advisor) before using any of the suggested remedies, techniques, or information in this book.

Upon using the contents and information contained in this book, you agree to hold harmless the Author from and against any damages, costs, and expenses, including any legal fees potentially resulting from the application of any of the information provided by this book. This disclaimer applies to any loss, damages or injury caused by the use and application, whether directly or indirectly, of any advice or information presented, whether for breach of contract, tort, negligence, personal injury, criminal intent, or under any other cause of action. You agree to accept all risks of using the information presented inside this book.

You agree that by continuing to read this book, where appropriate and/or necessary, you shall consult a professional (including but not limited to your doctor, attorney, or financial advisor or such other advisor as needed) before using any of the suggested remedies, techniques, or information in this book.

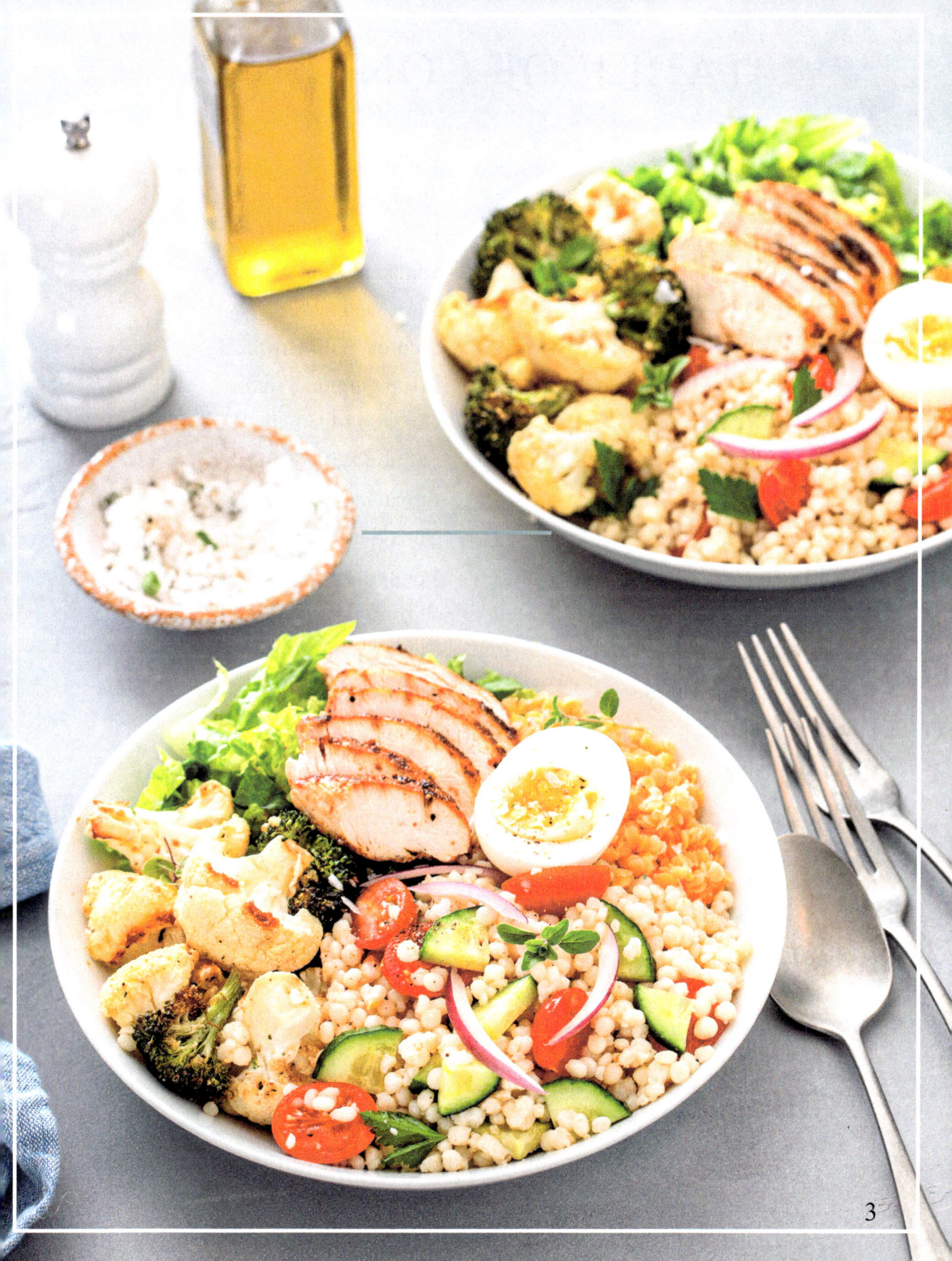

TABLE OF CONTENTS

DESCRIPTION	6
THE MIND DIET AND ITS IMPORTANCE FOR SENIORS	8
CORE PRINCIPLES OF THE MIND DIET FOR BRAIN HEALTH	12
FOODS TO INCLUDE AND LIMIT ON THE MIND DIET	16
HEALTHY HABITS AND TIPS FOR BRAIN HEALTH	20
BREAKFAST RECIPES	23
Avocado And Spinach Egg Toast	25
Oatmeal With Berries	27
Spiced Tofu & Cilantro Toast	29
Burrito With Vegetables	31
Spinach Smoothie	32
Quinoa Breakfast Bowl	33
Tomato & Leek Omelet	35
Sautéed Cabbage With Fried Egg	37
Broccoli Frittata	39
Scrambled Eggs With Asparagus & Green Peas	41
Avocado Egg Boats	43
Vegetable And Salmon Omelette	45
MAIN DISH	47
Fish With Vegetables	49
Quinoa Stuffed Bell Peppers	51
Anchovy Salad With Egg And Cherry Tomatoes	53
Chicken Chickpea Soup With Vegetables	54
Salmon With Broccoli	57
Fresh Quinoa Salad	59
Chicken Meatballs With Zucchini	61
Salmon With Spinach	62
Spinach And Berry Salad	63
Tuna Salad With Spinach	65
Lemon Herb Baked Chicken	67
Shrimp Power Bowl	68
Summer Quinoa Salad	71
Baked Salmon With Lemon And Herbs	73
Spinach And Broccoli Soup	75
Baked Salmon With Green Beans	77
Eggplant Melange	78
Carrot & Almond Salad	80
Radish & Avocado Salad	81
Veggie Roast	83
Grilled Shrimp Skewers	85
Chicken Patties	87
Chicken Meatball Soup	88
Chicken With Vegetables	91
Quinoa Veggie Patties	93

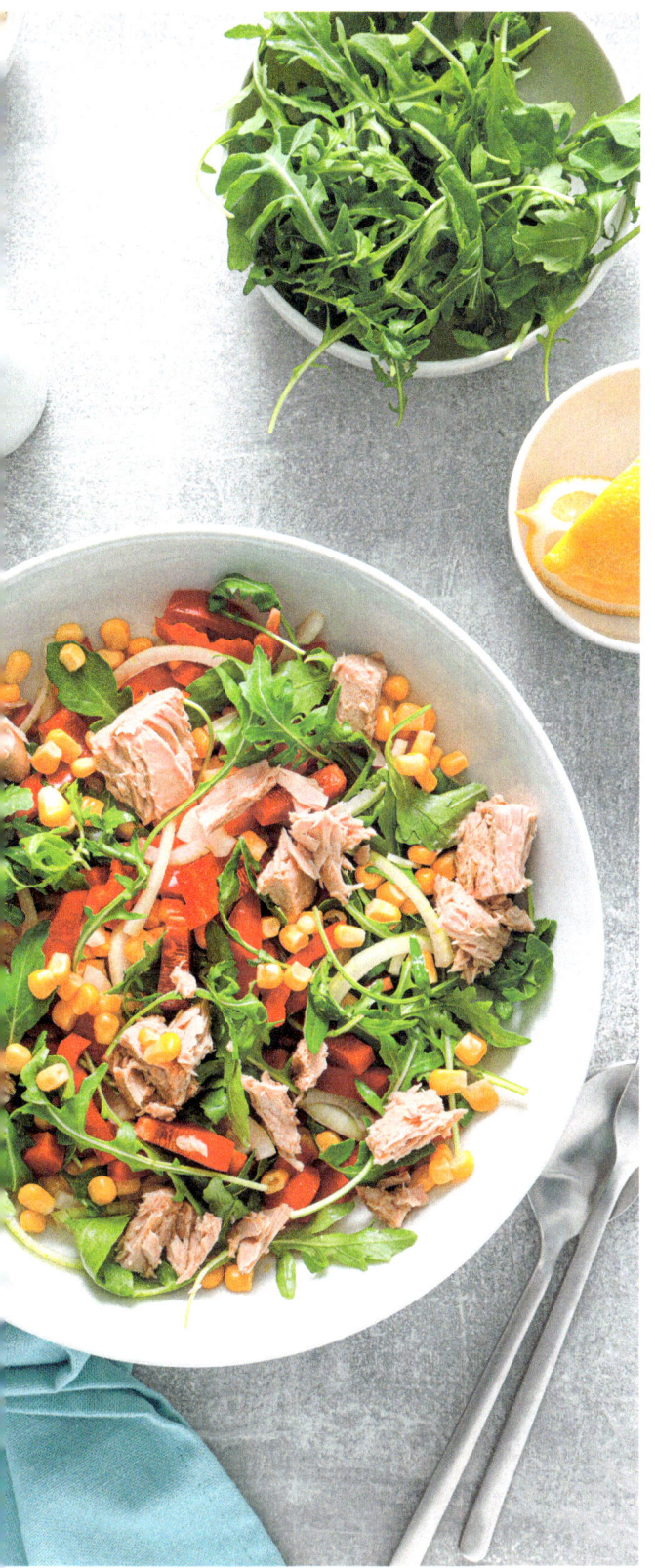

Turkey Meatballs With Mint	95
Steamed White Fish With Tomatoes	97
Chickpea Salad	98
Apple Spinach Salad	99
Aromatic Chicken Thighs With Herbs	101
Avocado, Cherry Tomato, Shrimp, And Arugula Salad	103

SNACKS & DESSERTS	105
Carrot And Red Cabbage Salad	107
Asparagus Spears	109
Roasted Broccoli Florets	111
Beetroot Chips	113
Broccoli Hummus	115
Panna Cotta With Strawberry Compote	117
Apple Chips	119
Strawberry Smoothie	120
Berry Smoothie	121
Cinnamon Peach Slices	123
Carrot Chips	125
Roasted Sweet Potato	127

CONCLUSION	128

DESCRIPTION

Aging gracefully means prioritizing brain health and maintaining cognitive function. The MIND diet (Mediterranean-DASH Intervention for Neurodegenerative Delay) is specially designed to support brain health and prevent cognitive decline. This cookbook, crafted with the needs of seniors in mind, offers simple, flavorful, and nourishing recipes that help you maintain mental clarity, improve memory, and protect your brain as you age.

«MIND Diet Cookbook for Seniors» is more than just a recipe collection. Inside, you'll find:

- A comprehensive guide to the MIND diet: Learn about the best foods for brain health and those to avoid.
- Lifestyle tips for holistic well-being: From nutrition and physical activity to cognitive exercises and sleep improvement.
- Step-by-step recipes tailored for easy preparation, considering seniors' taste preferences and dietary needs.

This book is your trusted guide to brain health, clear thinking, and an active, joyful life. Whether you're new to healthy eating or already focused on nutrition, «MIND Diet Cookbook for Seniors» will inspire you to make delicious, beneficial choices and turn each meal into a step toward enhanced well-being.

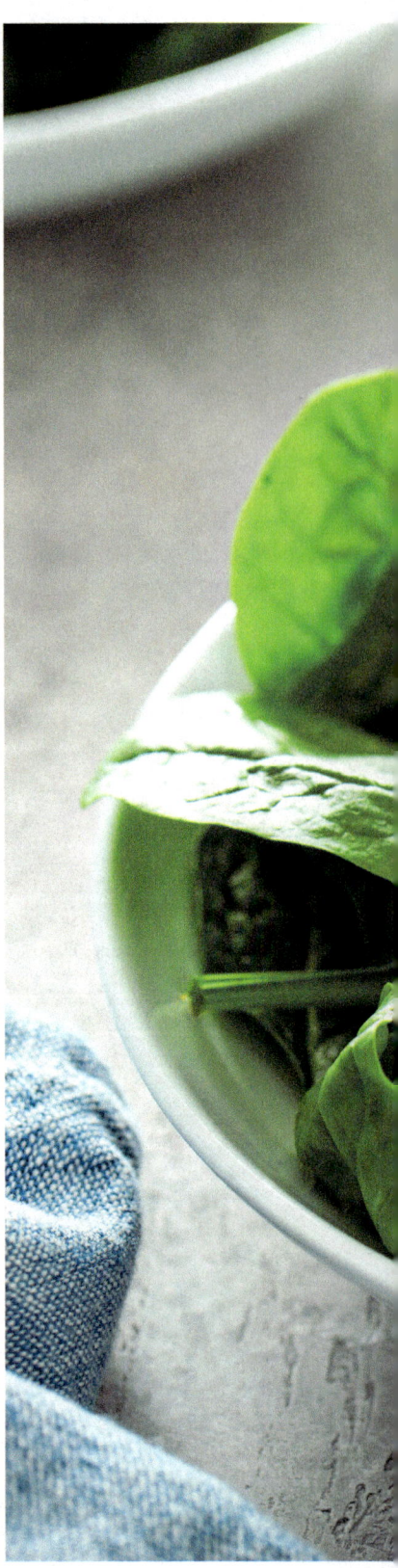

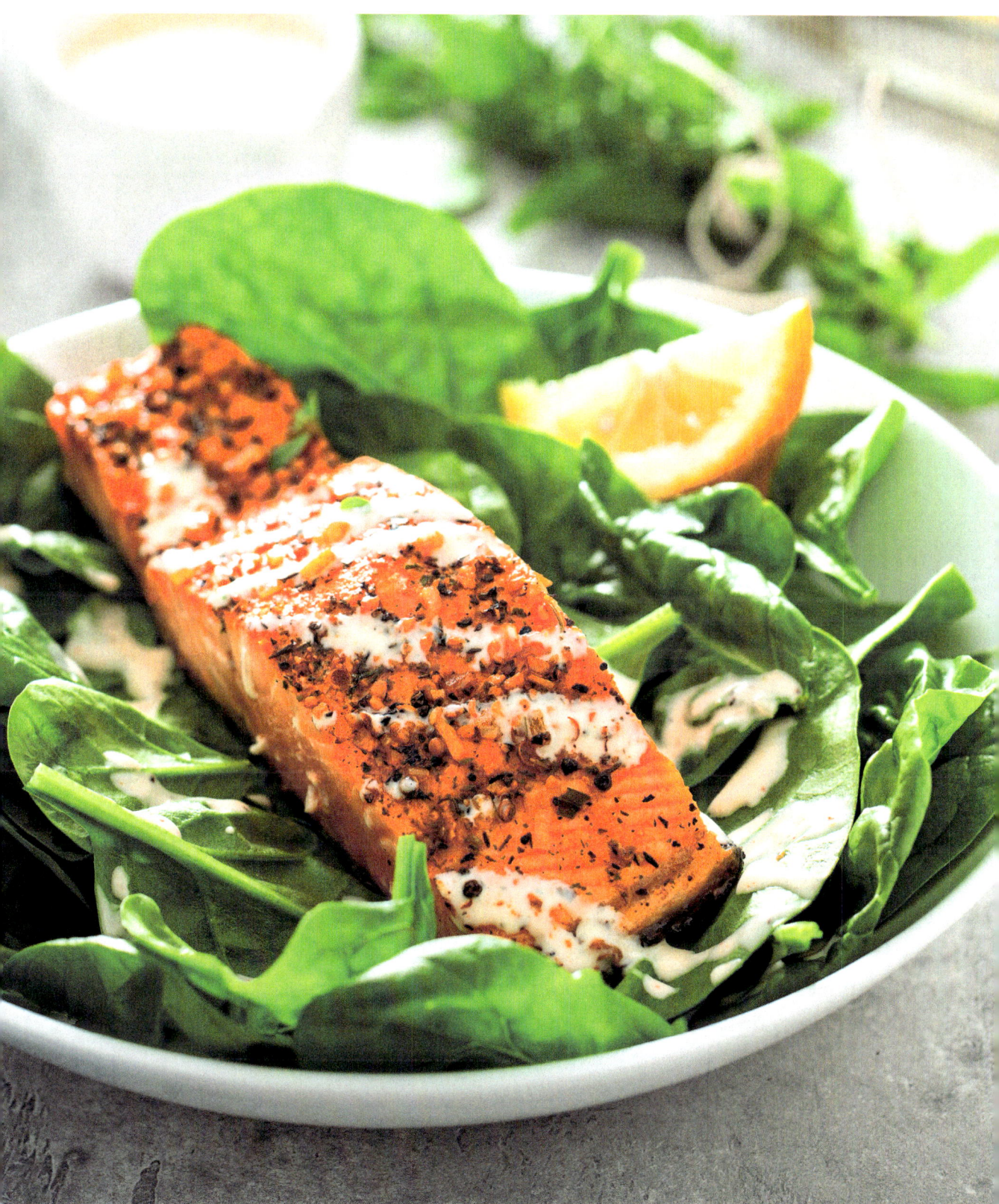

THE MIND DIET AND ITS IMPORTANCE FOR SENIORS

What is the MIND Diet?

The MIND diet, or Mediterranean-DASH Intervention for Neurodegenerative Delay, is a unique eating plan designed to improve brain health and slow cognitive aging. Combining principles from both the Mediterranean diet and the DASH diet — two of the world's most highly regarded dietary approaches for cardiovascular health — the MIND diet focuses on foods that support cognitive function and protect the brain from age-related changes. This diet highlights 10 specific food groups that nourish the brain and reduce the risk of neurodegenerative diseases, while recommending limits on 5 food categories that may negatively impact cognitive health.

The primary goal of the MIND diet is not only to reduce the risk of diseases like Alzheimer's but also to support memory, focus, and learning ability. The 10 brain-boosting food groups include leafy greens, berries, whole grains, nuts, fish, beans, and more, while foods like red meat, butter, cheese, sweets, and fried items are limited due to potential negative effects on brain health.

Scientific research provides robust support for the MIND diet's effectiveness in enhancing cognitive function through nutrients that reduce inflammation and oxidative stress — two significant contributors to age-related cognitive decline. Research led by Rush University Medical Center has shown that following the MIND diet can lower the risk of Alzheimer's disease by up to 53% with strict adherence, and even moderate adherence provides a 35% reduction in risk.

The main cognitive health benefits of the MIND diet include:

Protection from Inflammation and Oxidative Stress: Nutrients such as vitamin E and flavonoids, found in nuts, berries, and leafy greens, help neutralize free radicals that can harm brain cells.

Support for Neural Connectivity and Cognitive Function: Omega-3 fatty acids, especially abundant in fish, enhance cell membrane health and support effective neuron function.

Enhanced Memory and Focus: Antioxidant-rich foods like greens and berries improve blood flow, ensuring the brain receives enough oxygen for peak function.

Health Benefits of the MIND Diet

Improved Cognitive Function
One of the most significant advantages of the MIND diet is its ability to enhance cognitive function. Research shows that regularly consuming foods rich in antioxidants and healthy fats can support brain health, improve memory, and slow the progression of age-related changes.

Prevention of Brain Diseases
The MIND diet actively promotes the prevention of neurodegenerative diseases, such as Alzheimer's disease. Studies indicate that strict adherence to the diet's principles can reduce the risk by 53% for those who follow the recommendations closely and by 35% for those who do so moderately.

Support for Cardiovascular Health
Many of the foods included in the MIND diet help lower cholesterol levels and blood pressure, positively impacting cardiovascular health. A healthy heart ensures good blood flow to the brain, which is critical for its functioning.

Reduction of Inflammatory Processes
The foods recommended in the MIND diet are rich in antioxidants that help reduce inflammation in the body. Chronic inflammation is linked to many diseases, including cardiovascular and neurodegenerative disorders. Protecting against inflammation contributes to overall health and well-being.

Weight Management

The MIND diet focuses on balanced nutrition and includes plenty of fiber and nutrients, which help manage weight. Maintaining a healthy weight is a key factor in reducing the risk of various diseases, including diabetes and cardiovascular conditions.

Improved Mood

Some studies suggest that a diet rich in fruits, vegetables, nuts, and fish may positively impact mood and mental health. These foods, containing omega-3 fatty acids and vitamins, can promote the production of neurotransmitters, such as serotonin, which help maintain a good mood.

The MIND diet offers a wide range of health benefits that can significantly improve quality of life, especially for seniors. By focusing on foods that enhance cognitive function and reduce the risk of brain diseases, this dietary approach creates a strong foundation for healthy aging. Its principles not only support brain health but also contribute to overall physical well-being. To maximize these benefits, it's important to integrate the MIND diet into daily routines and seek guidance from a healthcare provider or dietitian for a personalized approach.

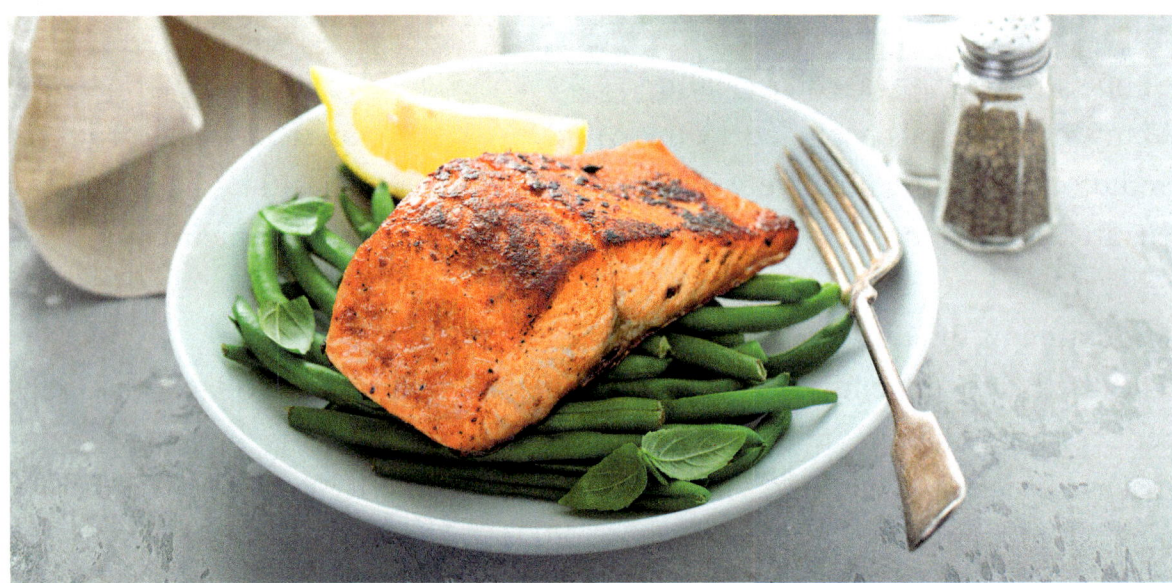

Why the MIND Diet is Important for Seniors

Aging brings natural changes to cognitive abilities such as memory, attention, and processing speed. For seniors, preserving brain health is essential to maintain independence, quality of life, and emotional well-being. The MIND diet addresses these age-related cognitive challenges, offering a nutritional strategy that can sustain and enhance mental clarity well into older adulthood. The MIND diet's brain-health benefits are particularly valuable for seniors, as research has shown it can reduce the risk of Alzheimer's and dementia significantly. Additionally, it fosters a lifestyle that values balanced nutrition, physical activity, and mental engagement. By focusing on nutrient-dense foods — especially those high in antioxidants, vitamins, and omega-3s — seniors can combat oxidative stress and inflammation, two significant contributors to cognitive aging. Foods like leafy greens, berries, and whole grains deliver the nutrients necessary to shield the brain from cellular damage, while reducing foods high in saturated fats and added sugars helps protect against cognitive decline. For seniors, the MIND diet is not just a way of eating but a holistic approach that promotes overall quality of life. Adopting this diet allows older adults to stay active, mentally engaged, and physically energized, knowing they are making positive choices for long-term brain health.

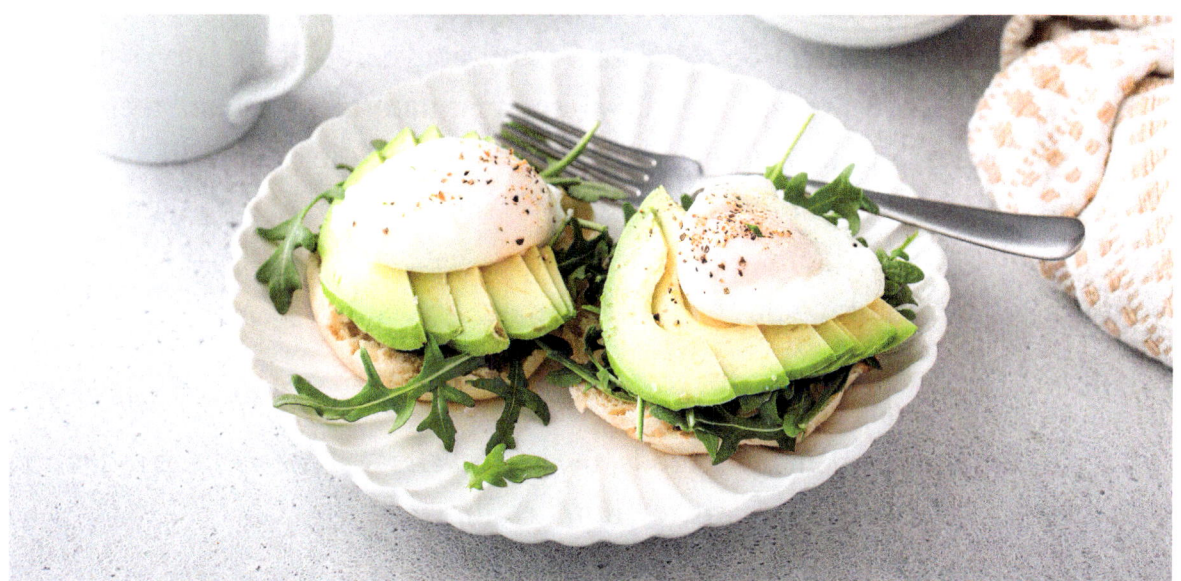

CORE PRINCIPLES OF THE MIND DIET FOR BRAIN HEALTH

In this chapter, we delve into the essential tenets of the MIND Diet and examine their profound significance for enhancing brain health. By understanding these core principles, you will gain insights into how specific dietary choices can foster cognitive function, protect against neurodegenerative diseases, and ultimately contribute to overall well-being.

Embrace Nutrient-Rich Foods
Central to the MIND Diet is a strong focus on whole, nutrient-dense foods that provide essential vitamins, minerals, antioxidants, and healthy fats. Key staples include leafy greens, berries, nuts, seeds, fish, whole grains, and olive oil. These foods are selected for their cognitive-enhancing properties and their protective effects against neurodegenerative diseases, making them ideal for seniors seeking to maintain their mental acuity.

Prioritize Brain-Boosting Nutrients
The MIND Diet highlights the importance of nutrients known to bolster brain health and cognitive function. Omega-3 fatty acids, found in fatty fish such as salmon and in walnuts, are crucial for maintaining neuronal membrane integrity and facilitating neurotransmitter activity. Antioxidants like vitamin E, vitamin C, and flavonoids help shield neurons from oxidative damage and inflammation, while vitamins B6, B12, and folate are vital for synthesizing neurotransmitters and regulating homocysteine levels.

Limit Harmful Foods
Alongside promoting beneficial foods, the MIND Diet encourages the reduction of substances that could jeopardize brain health.

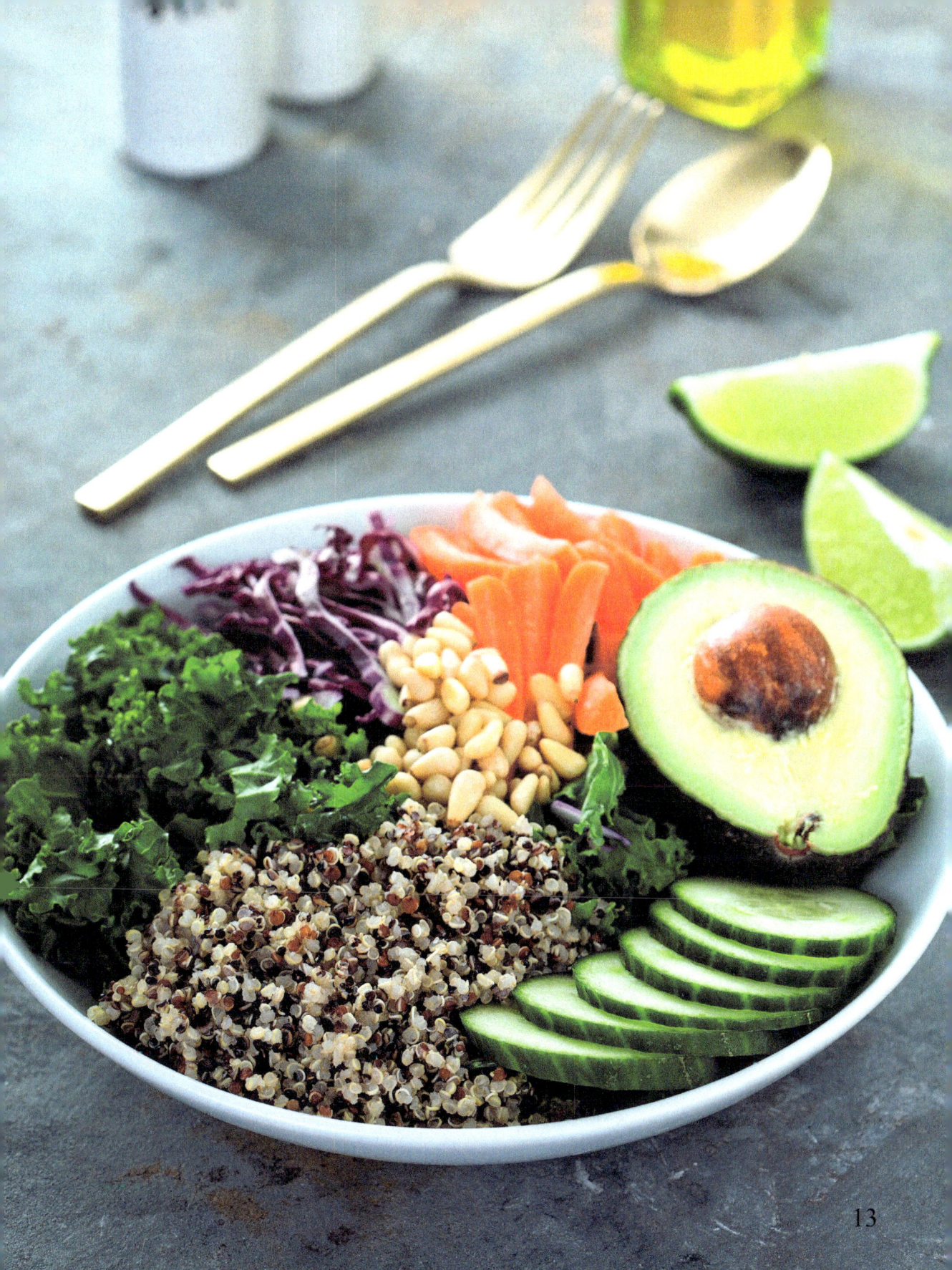

Processed foods high in refined sugars, saturated fats, and trans fats are discouraged, as they contribute to inflammation, insulin resistance, and oxidative stress — all factors linked to cognitive decline and neurodegenerative disorders.

Embrace Moderation and Balance
While the MIND Diet advocates for the inclusion of certain foods, moderation and balance remain pivotal in guiding dietary choices. Practicing portion control and mindful eating helps prevent the overconsumption of calorie-dense foods while ensuring a balanced intake of macronutrients. By achieving a harmonious balance between indulgence and restraint, seniors can enjoy a diverse and satisfying diet that supports their brain health.

Foster Consistency and Long-Term Commitment
The MIND Diet is not a temporary trend but a sustainable lifestyle choice aimed at promoting lifelong brain health. Consistency and long-term adherence to its principles are vital for fully realizing its benefits. By seamlessly incorporating the MIND Diet into their daily routines and making informed dietary choices, individuals can nourish their brains and protect their cognitive function well into the future.

In conclusion, the MIND Diet presents a comprehensive framework for enhancing brain health through nutrition, emphasizing the consumption of nutrient-rich foods, the limitation of harmful substances, and the cultivation of moderation and balance. By adopting these fundamental principles, seniors can leverage the transformative power of diet to foster cognitive vitality and enhance their overall well-being.

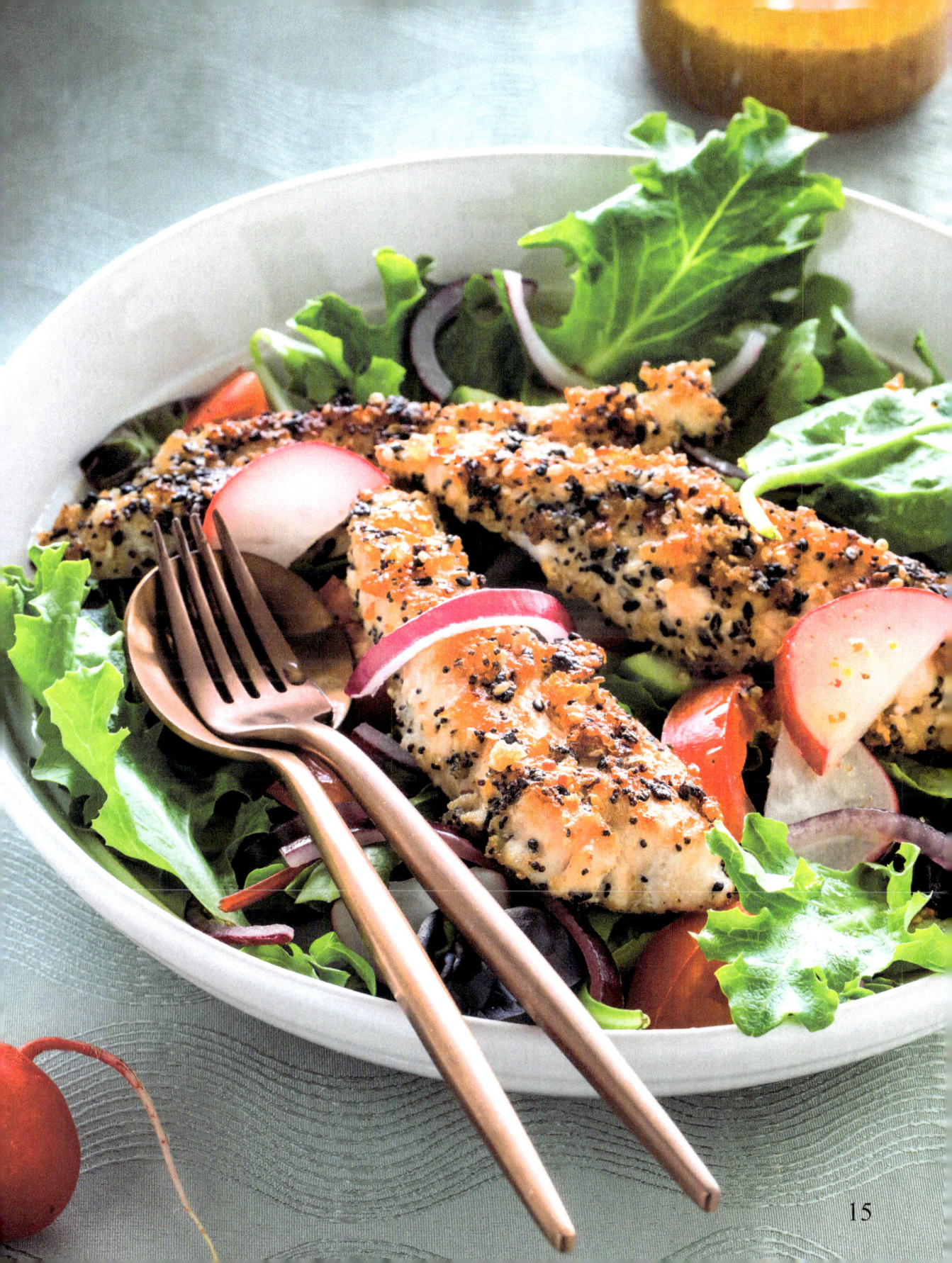

FOODS TO INCLUDE AND LIMIT ON THE MIND DIET

The MIND Diet is not just a collection of foods; it is a structured approach to eating that emphasizes specific food groups known for their cognitive benefits. Understanding which foods to embrace and which to limit is crucial for reaping the full benefits of this diet. In this chapter, we will outline the key foods to include in your meals and those to avoid, providing you with a clear roadmap for supporting your brain health.

Foods to Include:

Leafy Green Vegetables
Leafy greens such as spinach, kale, and collard greens are packed with essential nutrients, including vitamins A, C, K, and various antioxidants. These nutrients help reduce inflammation and oxidative stress, both of which are linked to cognitive decline.

Berries
Berries, particularly blueberries and strawberries, are rich in antioxidants known as flavonoids. Research suggests that these compounds may improve communication between brain cells, enhance memory, and protect against neurodegenerative diseases.

Nuts
Nuts, especially walnuts, are an excellent source of healthy fats, vitamin E, and omega-3 fatty acids, all of which play key roles in supporting brain health. Regular nut consumption has been linked to improved cognitive function and a lower risk of Alzheimer's disease, as these nutrients help reduce inflammation and protect brain cells from oxidative stress.

Additionally, nuts are versatile and can be easily added to meals and snacks, making them a convenient choice for promoting long-term brain health.

Fish

Fatty fish like salmon, mackerel, and sardines are loaded with omega-3 fatty acids, which are vital for maintaining brain health. Omega-3s contribute to the formation of neuronal membranes and support overall cognitive function.

Whole Grains

Whole grains such as oats, brown rice, and quinoa provide complex carbohydrates that fuel the brain. They also contain fiber, which supports digestive health and helps maintain steady blood sugar levels.

Olive Oil

As the primary fat source in the MIND Diet, olive oil is rich in monounsaturated fats and antioxidants. It has been linked to reduced inflammation and improved cognitive health.

Beans

Beans, including black beans, lentils, and chickpeas, are high in fiber and protein, making them a great addition to the MIND Diet. They provide sustained energy and nutrients that support brain health.

Poultry

Lean sources of protein like chicken and turkey are included in the MIND Diet. They offer important amino acids necessary for neurotransmitter production, aiding in cognitive function.

Wine (in Moderation)

Moderate consumption of red wine has been associated with a lower risk of cognitive decline, likely due to its antioxidant content. However, it's important to limit intake to one glass per day.

Foods to Avoid or Limit:

Red Meat
While not entirely eliminated, red meat should be consumed in moderation due to its higher saturated fat content, which may contribute to cognitive decline when eaten in excess.

Butter and Margarine
These fats are high in unhealthy saturated fats and trans fats. It's advisable to replace them with healthier fats, such as olive oil or avocado, to support brain health.

Cheese
Although delicious, cheese can be high in saturated fats and sodium. It's best to limit cheese intake to occasional use.

Pastries and Sweets
Foods high in added sugars and refined carbohydrates can lead to inflammation and insulin resistance, both of which are linked to cognitive decline.

Fried or Fast Foods
These foods are often high in unhealthy fats, sugars, and calories, which can negatively impact overall health and cognitive function. Opt for baked, grilled, or steamed options instead.

Adopting the MIND Diet means focusing on a variety of nutrient-rich foods while avoiding those that may harm brain health. Including recommended foods and limiting unhealthy ones can support cognitive function and long-term brain wellness. It's essential, however, to consult a healthcare professional or dietitian when making dietary changes. They can help create a personalized plan that fits your health needs, considering any allergies or intolerances. By working with a professional, you can ensure that your diet is both beneficial for brain health and tailored safely for you.

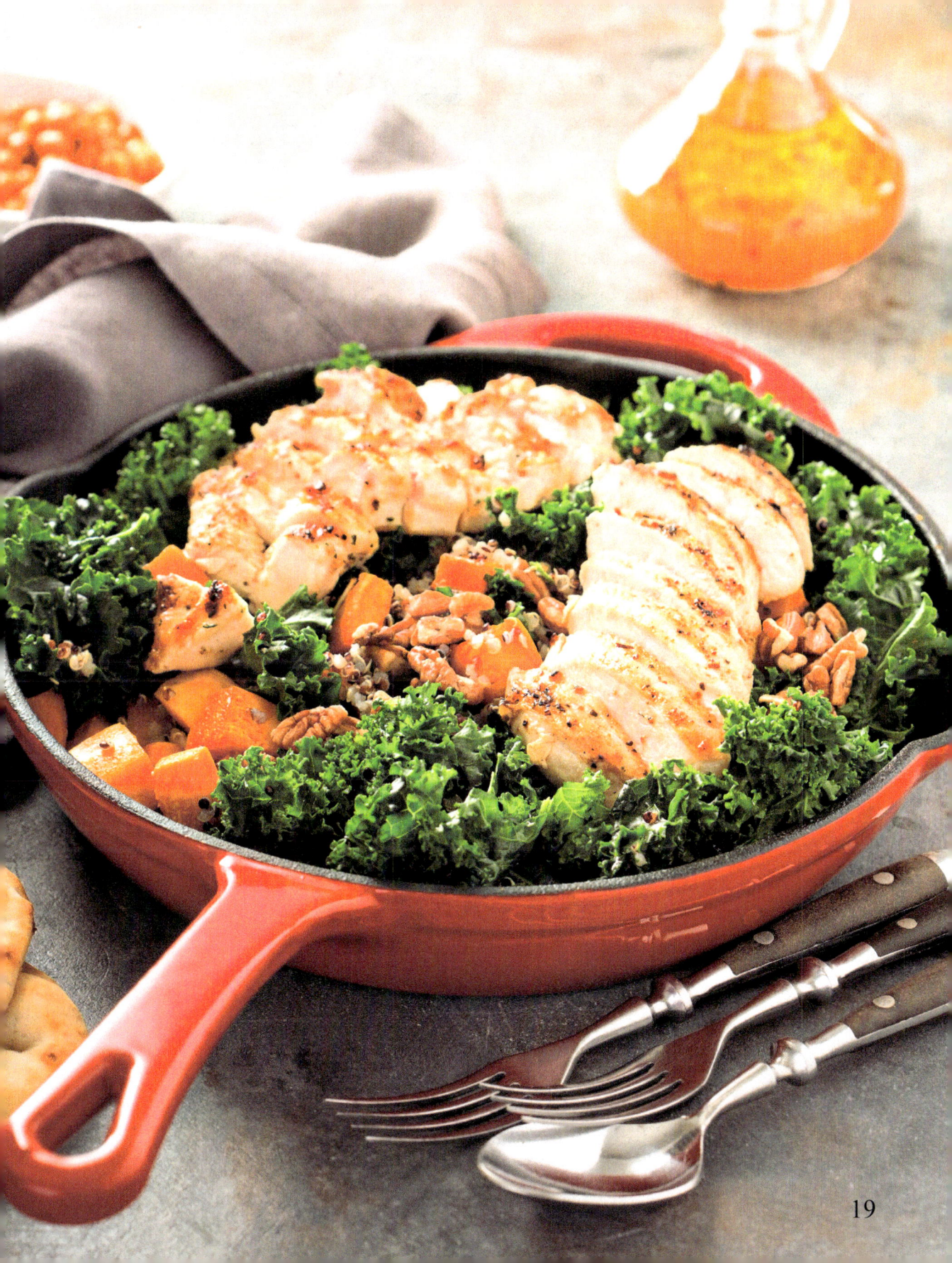

HEALTHY HABITS AND TIPS FOR BRAIN HEALTH

Maintaining brain health goes beyond just dietary choices; it encompasses a holistic approach that includes lifestyle habits and practices. This chapter outlines essential habits and practical tips that can support cognitive function and overall brain health as you age.

Stay Physically Active
Regular physical activity is crucial for brain health. Engaging in aerobic exercises, such as walking, jogging, swimming, or dancing, promotes blood flow to the brain, stimulates the growth of new neurons, and enhances cognitive function. Aim for at least 150 minutes of moderate aerobic activity each week, combined with strength training exercises on two or more days.

Prioritize Mental Stimulation
Challenging your brain is key to maintaining cognitive function. Engage in activities that stimulate your mind, such as puzzles, reading, learning a new language, or playing musical instruments. Consider taking up hobbies that require skill and focus, like knitting or woodworking. These activities can help build new neural connections and keep your brain sharp.

Foster Social Connections
Strong social ties can positively impact brain health. Stay connected with family and friends, join clubs or community groups, and participate in social activities. Engaging in conversations and shared experiences can help reduce feelings of isolation and depression, both of which can negatively affect cognitive function.

Get Quality Sleep
Sleep is vital for brain health. During sleep, the brain processes information, consolidates memories, and removes toxins.

Aim for 7-9 hours of quality sleep each night. Establish a regular sleep schedule, create a calming bedtime routine, and make your sleep environment comfortable and conducive to rest.

Manage Stress

Chronic stress can adversely affect brain health and cognitive function. Practice stress-reduction techniques such as mindfulness, meditation, yoga, or deep-breathing exercises. Engaging in regular physical activity and maintaining strong social connections can also help mitigate stress.

Stay Hydrated

Proper hydration is essential for optimal brain function. Dehydration can impair cognitive abilities and lead to fatigue and confusion. Aim to drink enough water throughout the day, and pay attention to signs of dehydration, such as dry mouth or decreased urine output.

Limit Alcohol Consumption

While moderate alcohol consumption may have some benefits for heart health, excessive drinking can lead to cognitive decline and increase the risk of neurodegenerative diseases. If you choose to drink, limit your intake to one drink per day for women and two drinks per day for men.

Consider Brain-Healthy Supplements

Certain supplements may support brain health, including omega-3 fatty acids, vitamin D, B vitamins, and antioxidants. Consult with your healthcare provider before starting any new supplements to ensure they are appropriate for you.

Incorporating these healthy habits and tips into your daily routine can significantly enhance brain health and cognitive function. By staying physically active, mentally engaged, socially connected, and mindful of your overall well-being, you can take proactive steps to support your brain health as you age. Remember, a holistic approach that combines a balanced diet, physical activity, mental stimulation, and healthy lifestyle choices is the key to maintaining cognitive vitality for years to come.

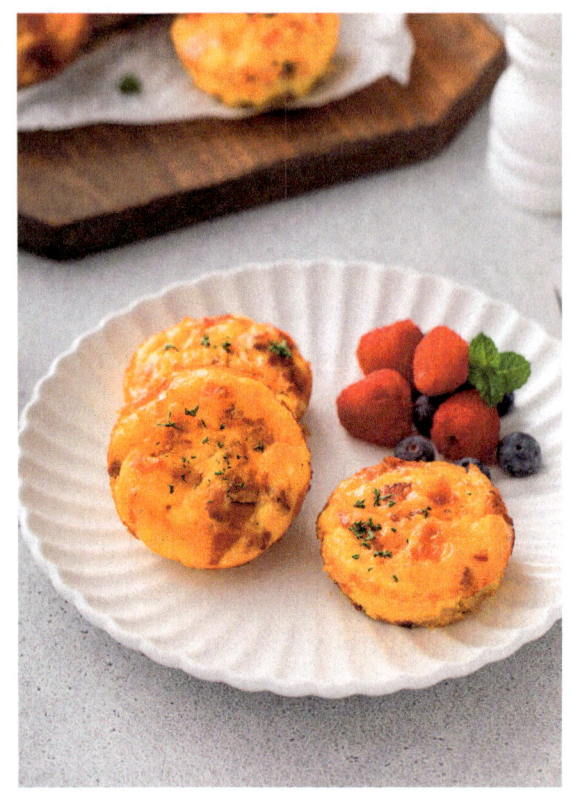
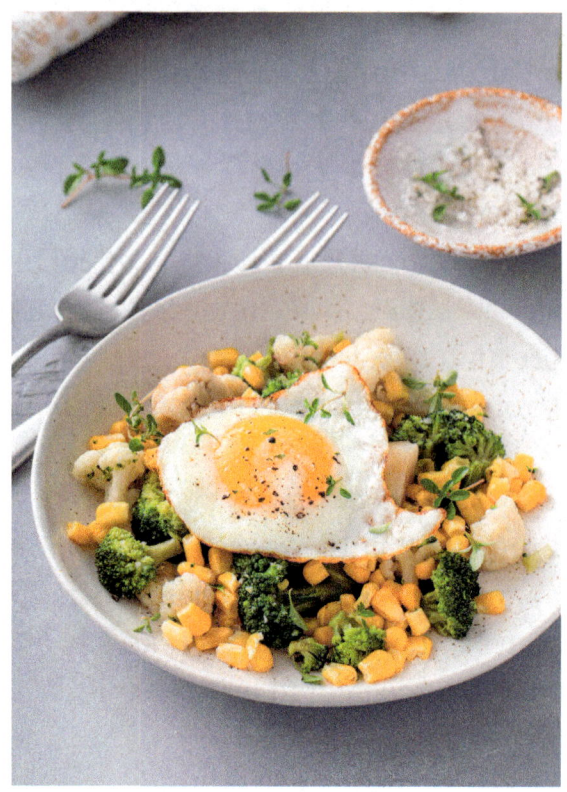
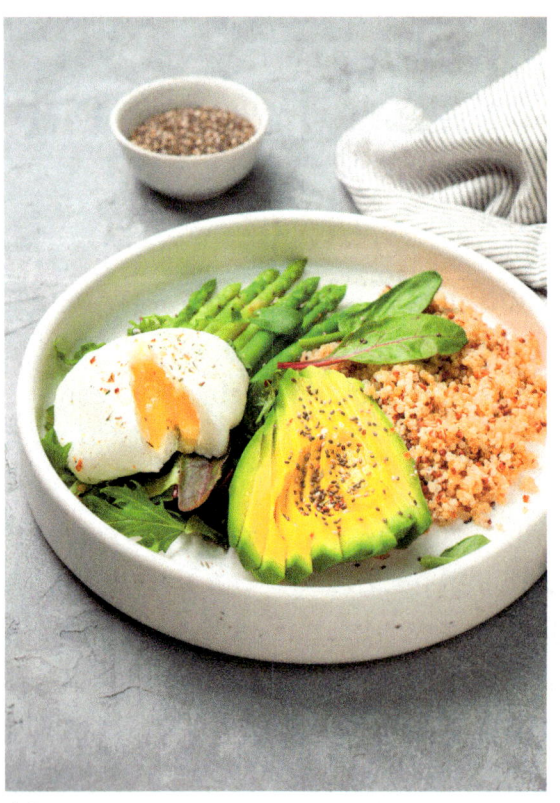
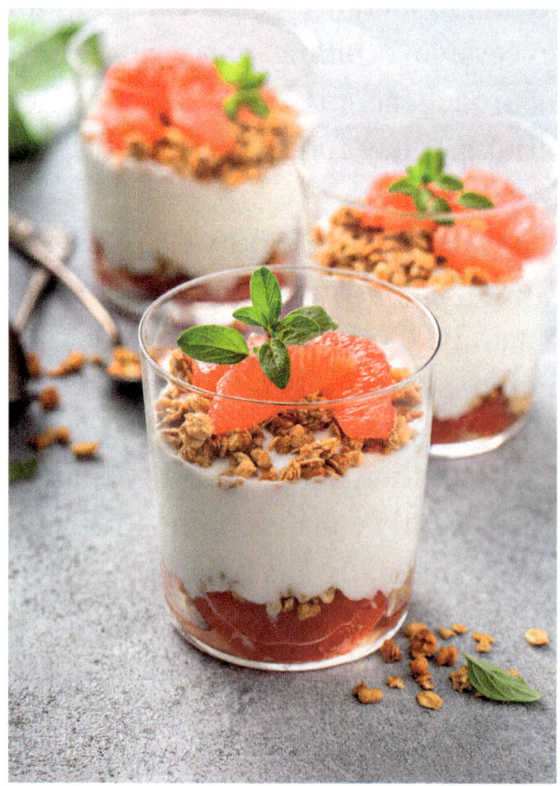

BREAKFAST RECIPES

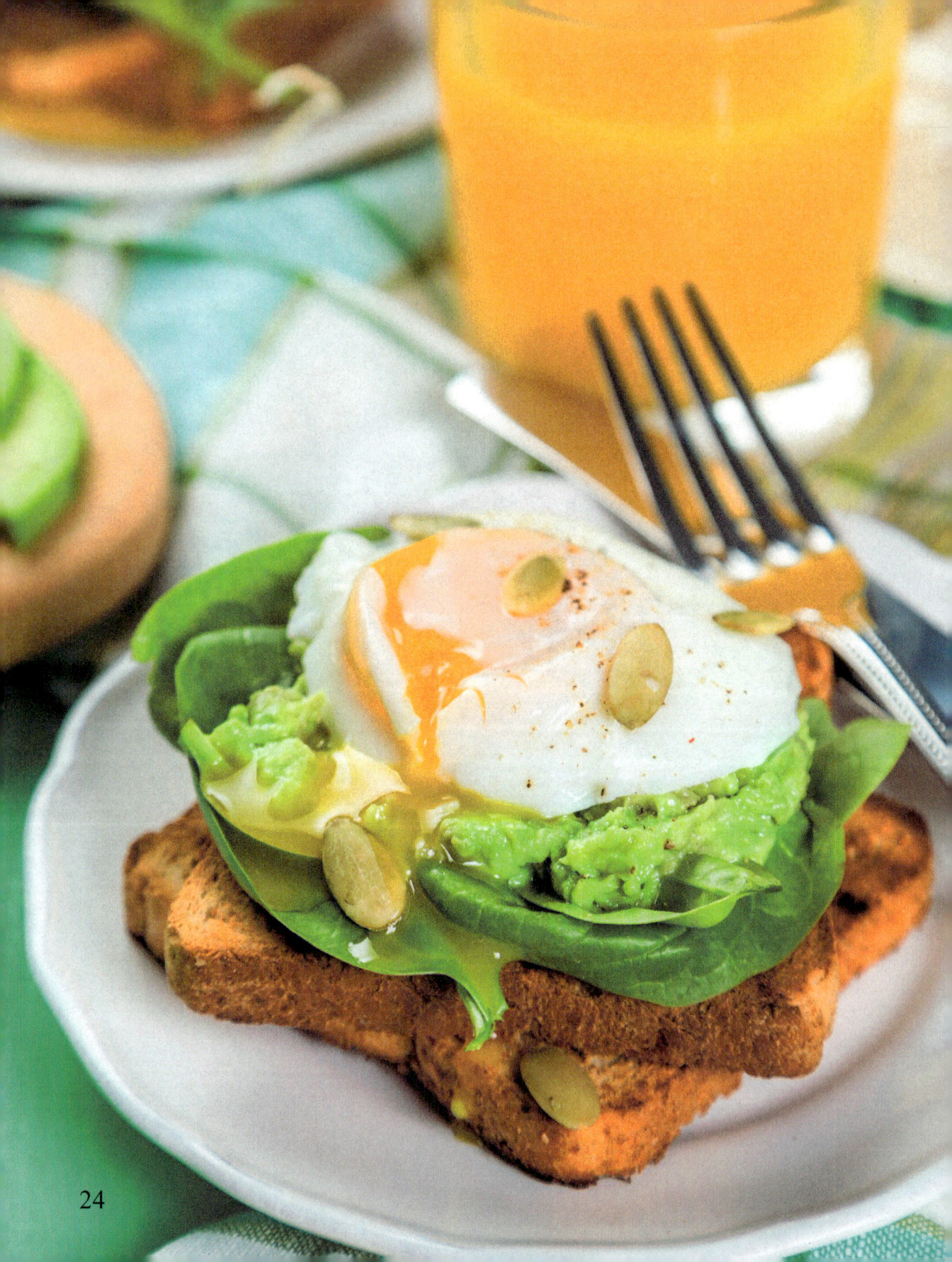

AVOCADO AND SPINACH EGG TOAST

 Cooking Difficulty: 2/10

 Cooking Time: 9 minutes

 Servings: 1

INGREDIENTS

- 1 slice whole grain bread
- 1/2 ripe avocado
- 1 cup fresh spinach leaves
- 1 large egg
- 1 tsp olive oil
- salt and pepper to taste
- optional: cherry tomatoes, a sprinkle of red pepper flakes, or a squeeze of lemon juice for extra flavor

DESCRIPTION

STEP 1
Toast the whole grain bread until crispy. Mash the avocado in a bowl with a pinch of salt and pepper.

STEP 2
Heat olive oil in a skillet over medium heat. Sauté spinach until wilted (2-3 minutes), then set aside. In the same skillet, cook the egg to your liking (sunny-side up, over-easy, or scrambled) and season with salt and pepper.

STEP 3
Spread the mashed avocado on the toasted bread. Top with sautéed spinach and the cooked egg.

NUTRITIONAL INFORMATION

169 Calories, 2.5g Fat, 4.4g Carbs, 3.1g Protein

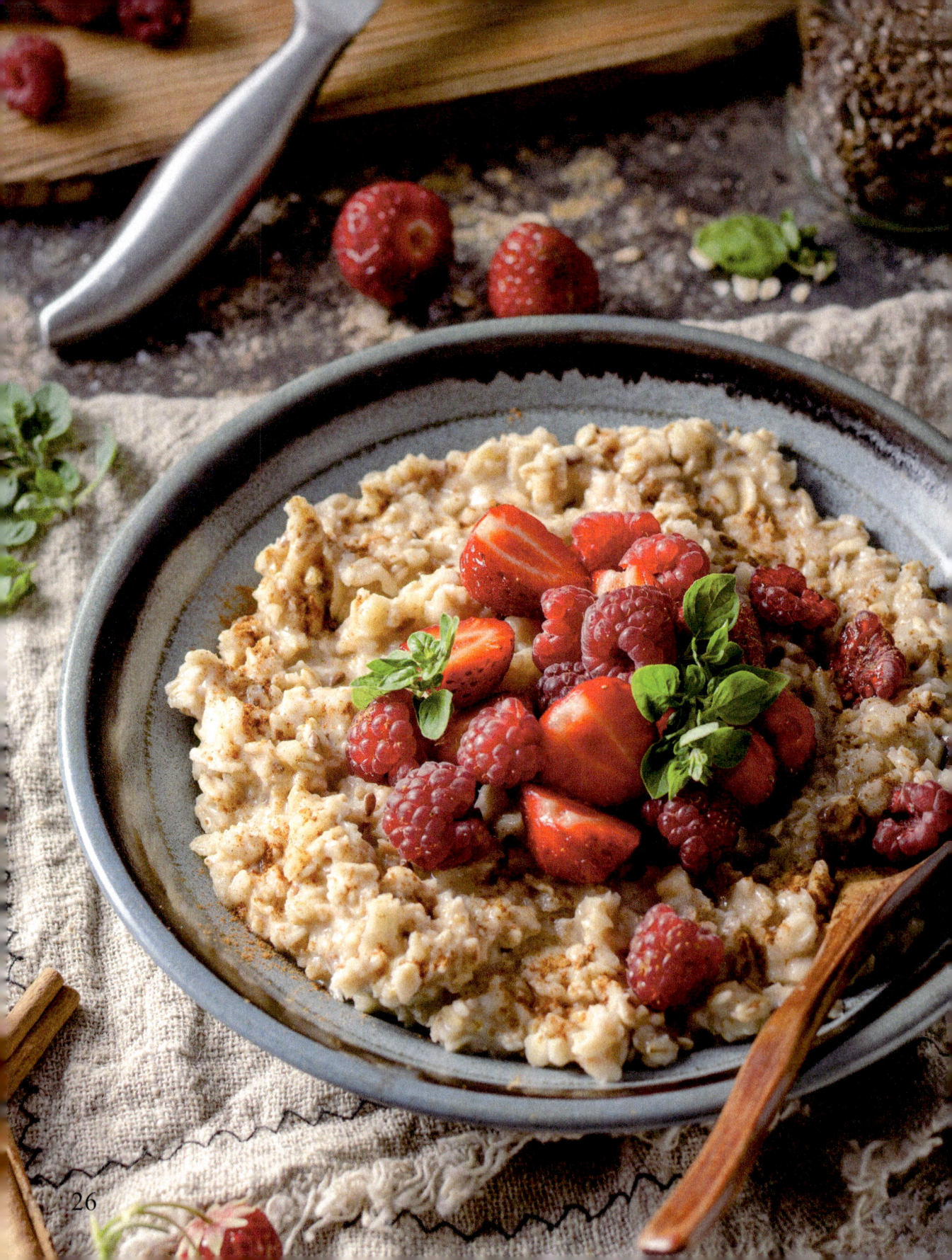

OATMEAL WITH BERRIES

 Cooking Difficulty: 1/10

 Cooking Time: 8 minutes

 Servings: 2

INGREDIENTS

- 1 cup rolled oats
- 2 cups unsweetened almond milk
- 1 tablespoon honey or maple syrup (optional)
- 1/2 teaspoon vanilla extract (optional)
- a pinch of salt
- 1/2 cup fresh raspberries
- 1/2 cup fresh strawberries, sliced
- 1 tablespoon chopped almonds (optional, for garnish)

DESCRIPTION

STEP 1
In a medium saucepan, combine oats, almond milk, honey or maple syrup (if using), vanilla extract, and salt. Bring the mixture to a gentle boil over medium heat, then reduce to low heat and simmer, stirring occasionally, for 5-7 minutes, or until the oats are soft and the oatmeal reaches your desired consistency. Remove from heat and divide the oatmeal between two bowls.

STEP 2
Top each bowl with fresh raspberries, sliced strawberries, and a sprinkle of chopped almonds if desired. Serve warm, and enjoy!

NUTRITIONAL INFORMATION
258 Calories, 8g Fat, 15g Carbs, 7g Protein

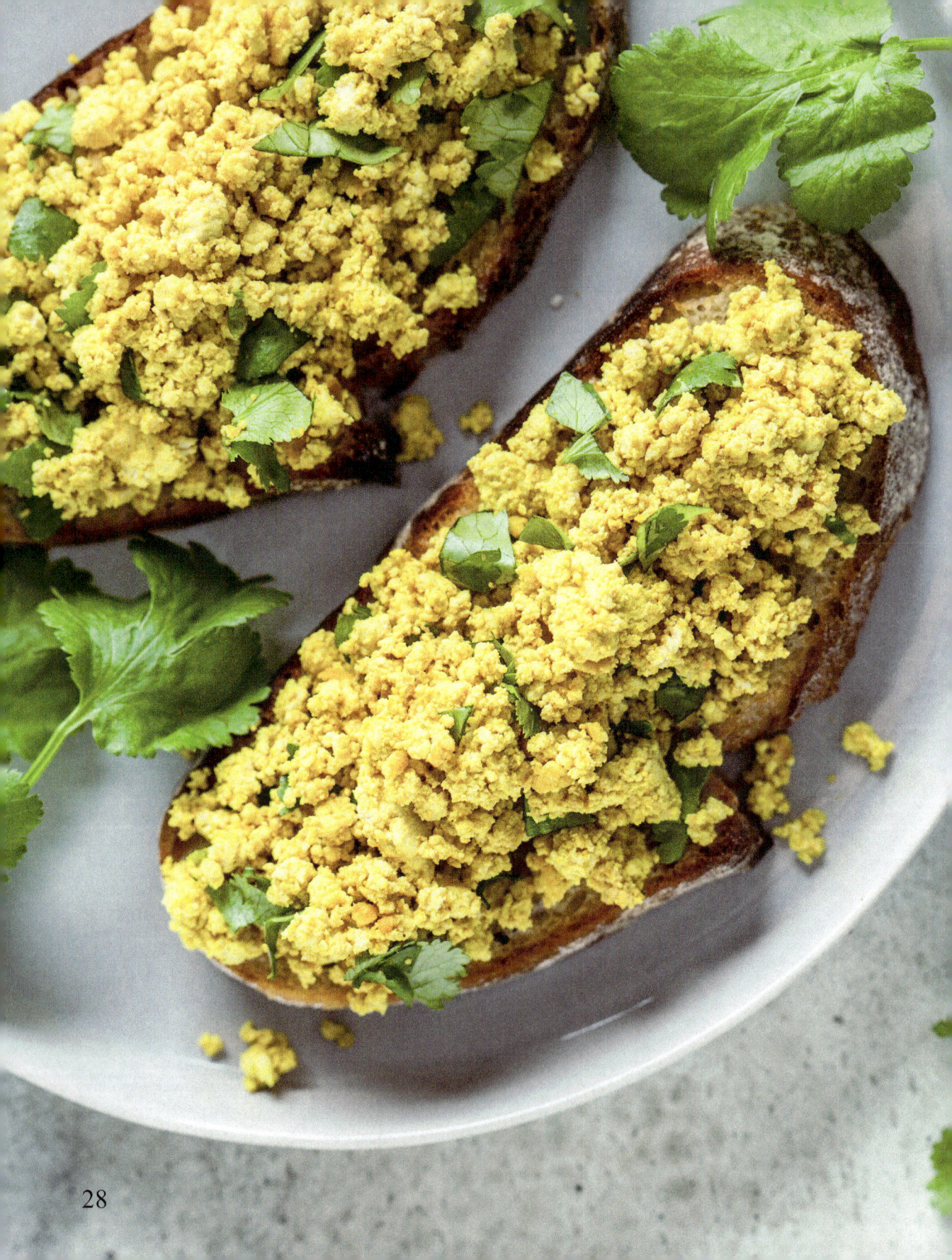

SPICED TOFU & CILANTRO TOAST

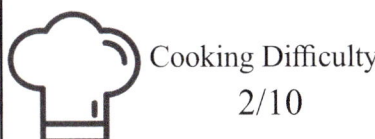 Cooking Difficulty: 2/10

 Cooking Time: 10 minutes

 Servings: 2

INGREDIENTS

- 4 slices whole grain bread
- 1/2 block firm tofu, patted dry and crumbled
- 1 tablespoon olive oil
- 1/2 teaspoon ground turmeric
- 1/2 teaspoon smoked paprika
- 1/4 teaspoon ground cumin
- 1/4 teaspoon garlic powder
- salt and pepper, to taste
- fresh cilantro, chopped, for garnish
- 1/2 avocado, sliced (optional)

DESCRIPTION

STEP 1
In a medium skillet, heat olive oil over medium heat. Add crumbled tofu, turmeric, smoked paprika, cumin, and garlic powder, stirring well to coat. Cook the tofu for 5-7 minutes, stirring occasionally, until lightly browned and fragrant. Season with salt and pepper to taste. While the tofu is cooking, toast the whole grain bread slices until golden.

STEP 2
Top each toast slice with the spiced tofu and garnish generously with fresh cilantro. Add sliced avocado if desired. Serve warm and enjoy!

NUTRITIONAL INFORMATION

200 Calories, 3g Fat, 27g Carbs, 5g Protein

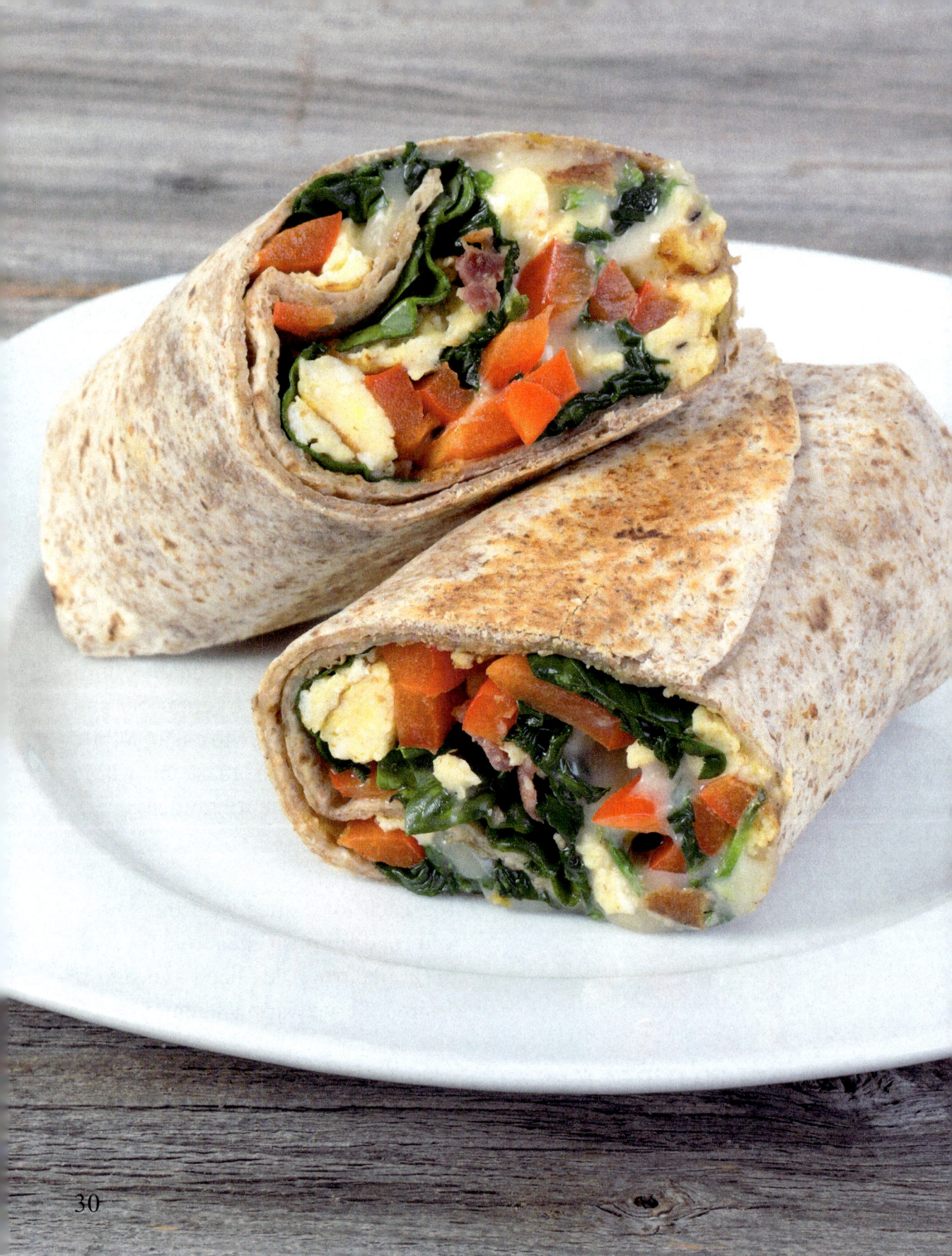

BURRITO WITH VEGETABLES

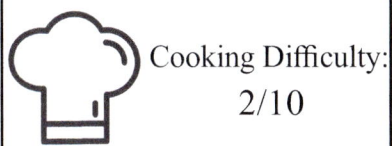 Cooking Difficulty: 2/10

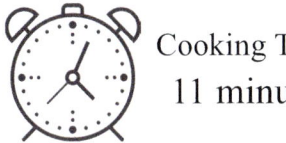 Cooking Time: 11 minutes

 Servings: 2

INGREDIENTS

- 4 eggs
- 4 large tortillas
- 1 red bell pepper, sliced
- 2 cups fresh spinach
- 2 small tomatoes, diced
- salt and pepper to taste
- olive oil for cooking

DESCRIPTION

STEP 1
In a large skillet, heat a little olive oil over medium heat. Add the red bell pepper to the skillet and cook, until softened, about 5 minutes. Add the fresh spinach to the skillet and cook 2-3 minutes. In a separate bowl, beat the eggs and season with salt and pepper to taste.

STEP 2
Add the beaten eggs to the skillet with the vegetables. Cook, stirring, until the eggs are cooked through. Divide the cooked vegetables and eggs evenly among each tortilla. Roll up the burritos, folding in the sides, to enclose the filling.

NUTRITIONAL INFORMATION
300 Calories, 15g Fat, 25g Carbs, 15g Protein

SPINACH SMOOTHIE

 Cooking Difficulty: 1/10	 Cooking Time: 11 minutes	 Servings: 1

INGREDIENTS

- 1 cup fresh spinach
- 1 ripe banana
- 1 cup unsweetened almond milk
- 1 tablespoon almond butter (optional)
- ice cubes (optional)

DESCRIPTION

STEP 1

In a blender, combine spinach, banana, almond milk, and almond butter. Blend until smooth. If desired, add ice cubes and blend again for a chilled smoothie. Pour into glasses and enjoy your healthy breakfast!

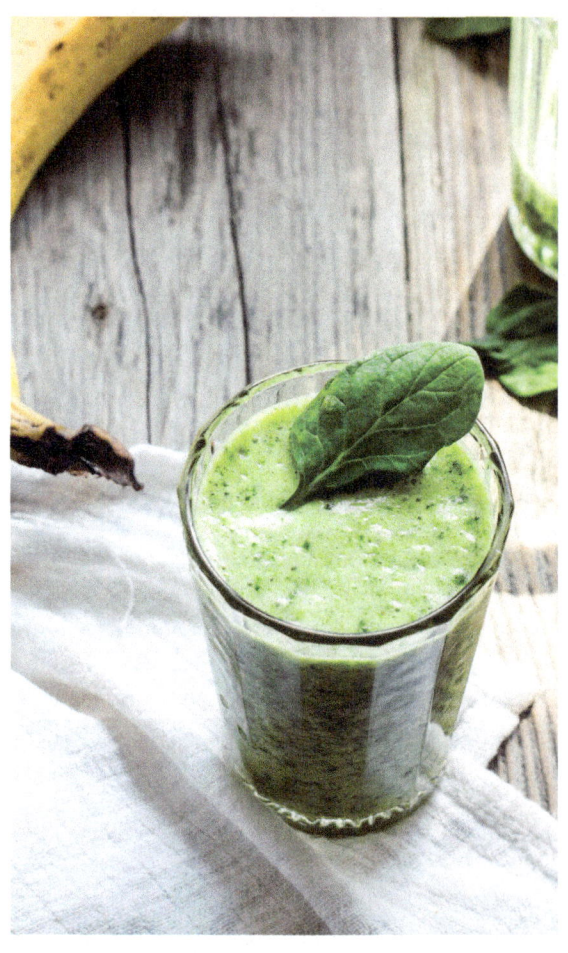

NUTRITIONAL INFORMATION

300 Calories, 15g Fat, 25g Carbs, 15g Protein

QUINOA BREAKFAST BOWL

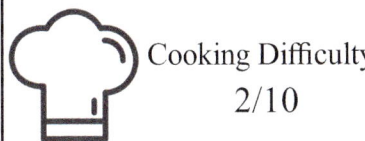 Cooking Difficulty: 2/10　 Cooking Time: 11 minutes　 Servings: 2

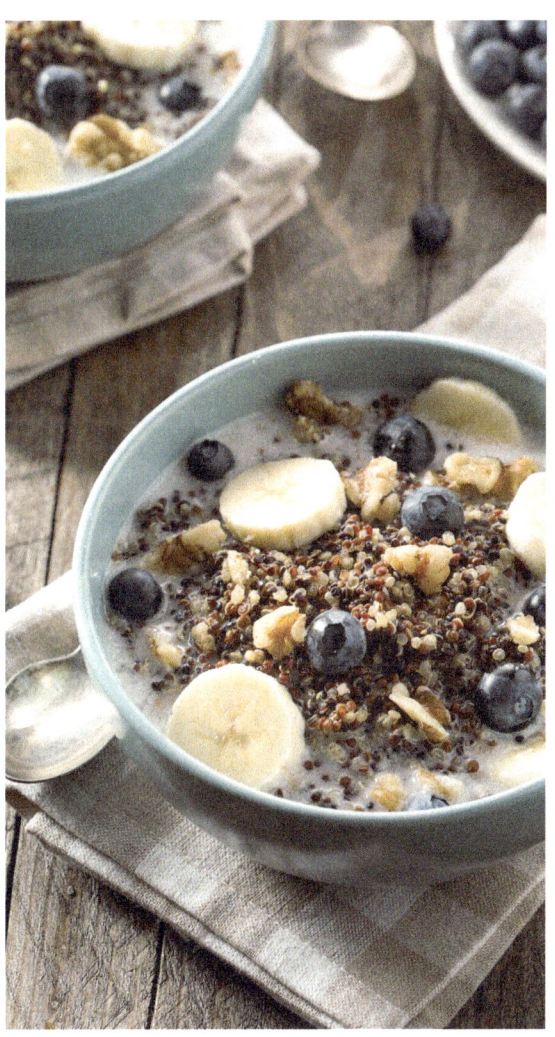

INGREDIENTS

- 1 cup cooked quinoa
- 1 cup almond milk
- 1/2 teaspoon cinnamon
- 1 tablespoon maple syrup (optional)
- 1/2 cup sliced bananas or berries
- 2 tablespoons chopped nuts

DESCRIPTION

STEP 1

In a saucepan, combine cooked quinoa, almond milk, cinnamon, and maple syrup. Heat over medium until warm. Spoon the warm quinoa into bowls and top with sliced bananas or berries and chopped nuts.

NUTRITIONAL INFORMATION

300 Calories, 15g Fat, 25g Carbs, 15g Protein

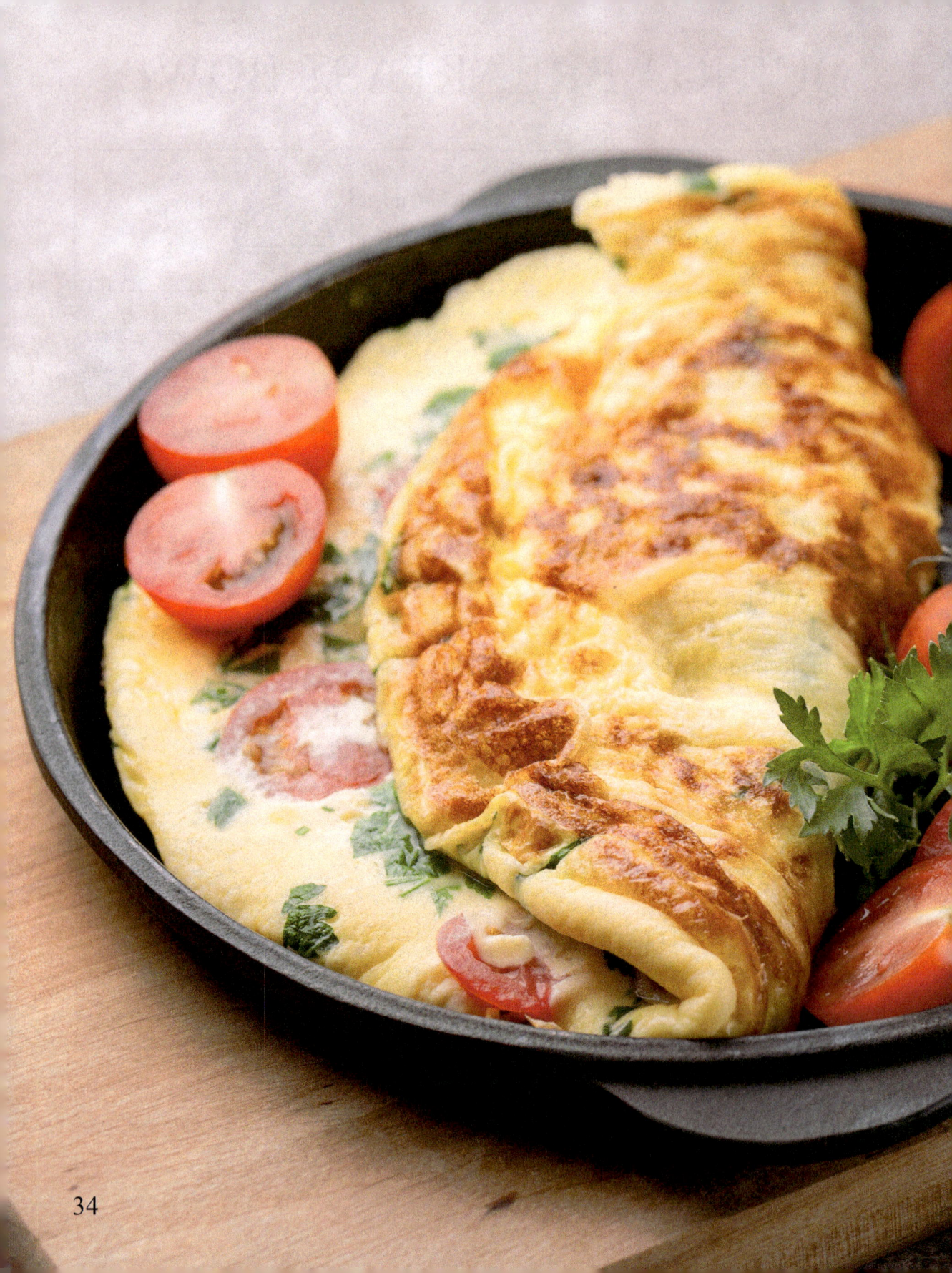

TOMATO & LEEK OMELET

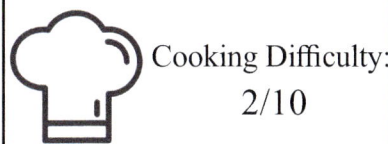 Cooking Difficulty: 2/10

 Cooking Time: 14 minutes

 Servings: 2

INGREDIENTS

- 2 large eggs (or 1/2 cup egg whites, if preferred)
- 2 tablespoons unsweetened almond milk
- salt and pepper, to taste
- 1/4 cup cherry tomatoes, halved
- 1/4 cup thinly sliced leeks (white and light green parts only)
- 1 tablespoon olive oil
- fresh parsley, chopped, for garnish

DESCRIPTION

STEP 1
In a bowl, whisk eggs, almond milk, salt, and pepper. Set aside. Heat olive oil in a nonstick skillet over medium heat. Add leeks, cooking for 2-3 minutes until softened. Add tomatoes and cook 1-2 more minutes.

STEP 2
Pour egg mixture over the vegetables. Cook for 3-4 minutes, stirring edges gently. Flip or fold in half, cooking another 1-2 minutes until set.

STEP 3
Transfer to a plate, garnish with parsley, and enjoy warm.

NUTRITIONAL INFORMATION
274 Calories, 11g Fat, 8g Carbs, 15g Protein

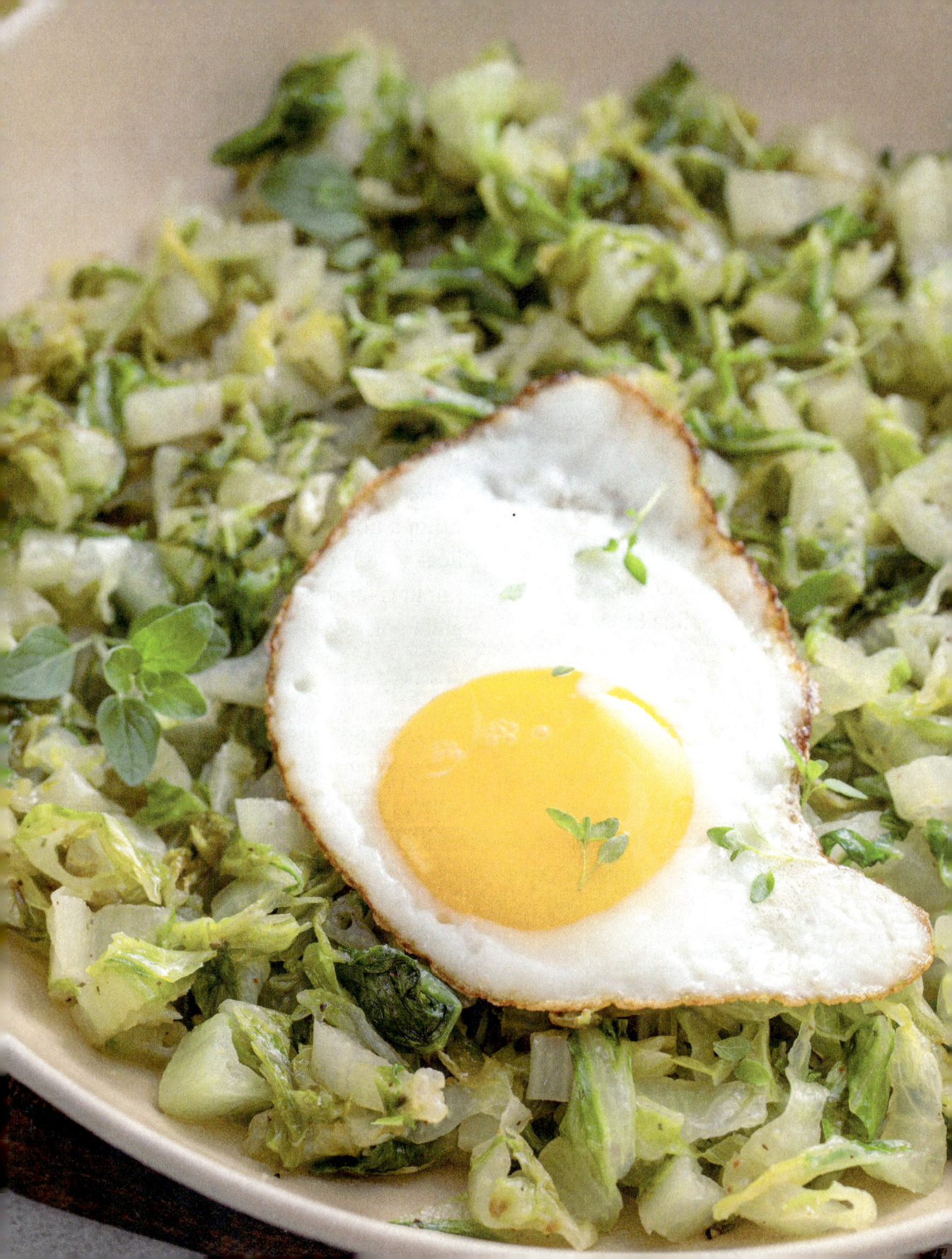

SAUTÉED CABBAGE WITH FRIED EGG

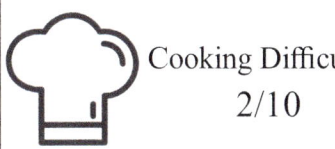 Cooking Difficulty: 2/10

 Cooking Time: 18 minutes

 Servings: 2

INGREDIENTS

- 2 cups shredded green cabbage
- 1 small onion, thinly sliced
- 2 tablespoons olive oil
- 1 teaspoon garlic powder
- 1/2 teaspoon smoked paprika
- salt and pepper, to taste
- 2 large eggs
- fresh parsley or chives, for garnish (optional)

DESCRIPTION

STEP 1
In a skillet, heat olive oil over medium heat. Add onion and sauté for 3-4 minutes. Stir in cabbage, garlic powder, smoked paprika, salt, and pepper, cooking for 8-10 minutes until tender.

STEP 2
In a separate skillet, fry the eggs to your liking.

STEP 3
Plate the sautéed cabbage and top with a fried egg. Garnish with fresh herbs, if desired. Enjoy!

NUTRITIONAL INFORMATION
146 Calories, 4g Fat, 5g Carbs, 5g Protein

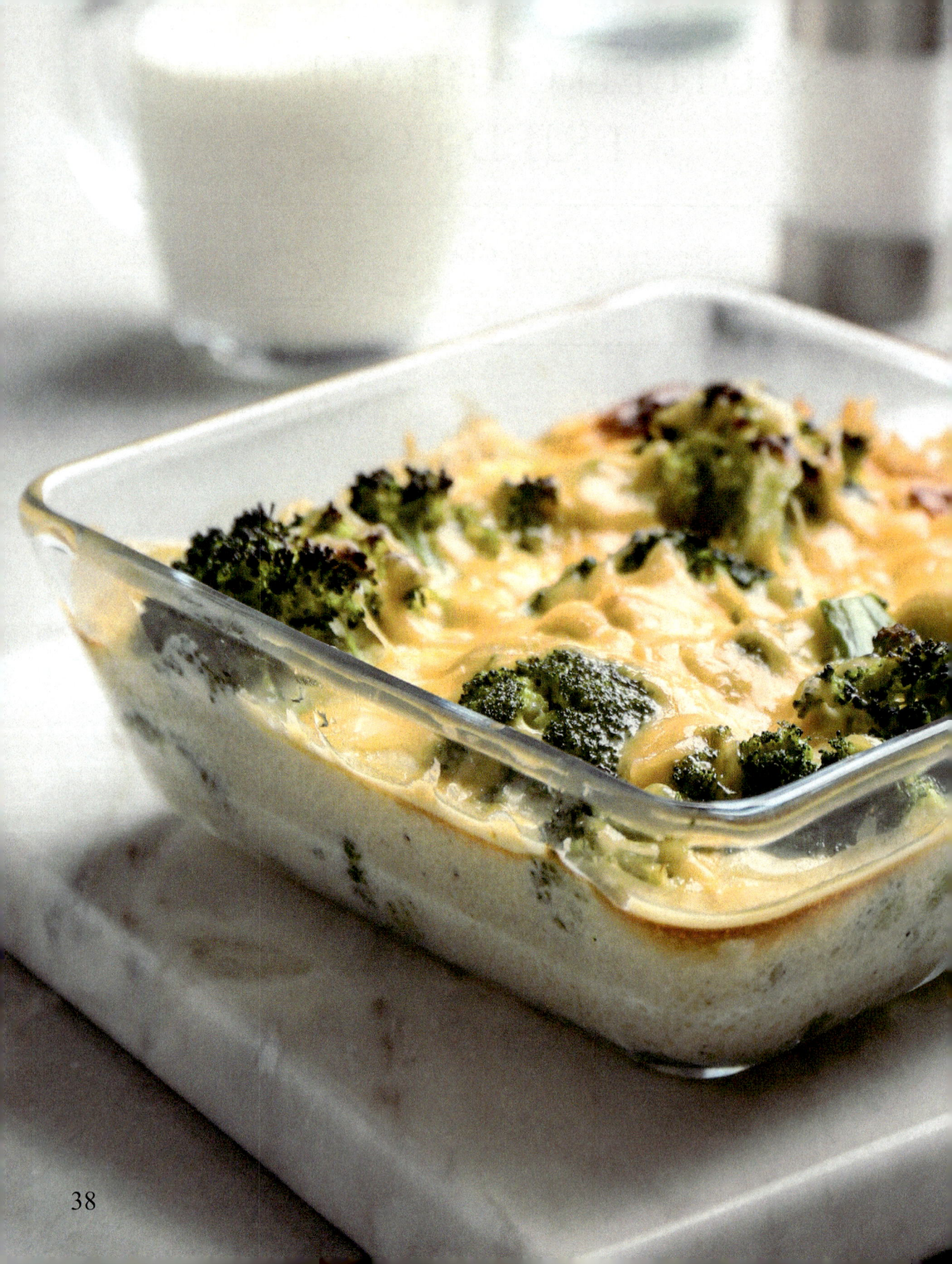

BROCCOLI FRITTATA

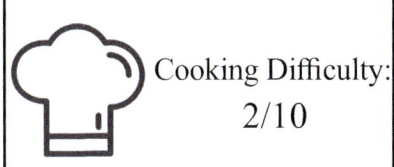 Cooking Difficulty: 2/10

 Cooking Time: 24 minutes

 Servings: 2

INGREDIENTS

- 3 eggs
- 1/2 cup unsweetened almond milk (or other plant milk)
- 1/2 cup broccoli florets
- 1/4 cup vegan shredded cheese
- 1 tablespoon olive oil
- salt and pepper, to taste
- 1/4 teaspoon turmeric (for color)
- 1/4 teaspoon garlic powder (optional, for flavor)

DESCRIPTION

STEP 1
Preheat oven to 350 degrees F (175 degrees C). Cut broccoli into florets and steam or boil in a pot of boiling water for 3-4 minutes.

STEP 2
In a bowl, whisk together eggs, almond milk, turmeric, garlic powder (if using), salt, and pepper until smooth. Heat olive oil in a nonstick, oven-safe skillet over medium heat. Add the steamed broccoli and cook for 2-3 minutes. Pour egg mixture over broccoli. Sprinkle with shredded cheese. Transfer skillet to oven and bake for 15-20 minutes, or until golden brown. Serve and enjoy!

NUTRITIONAL INFORMATION

250 Calories, 20g Fat, 5g Carbs, 15g Protein

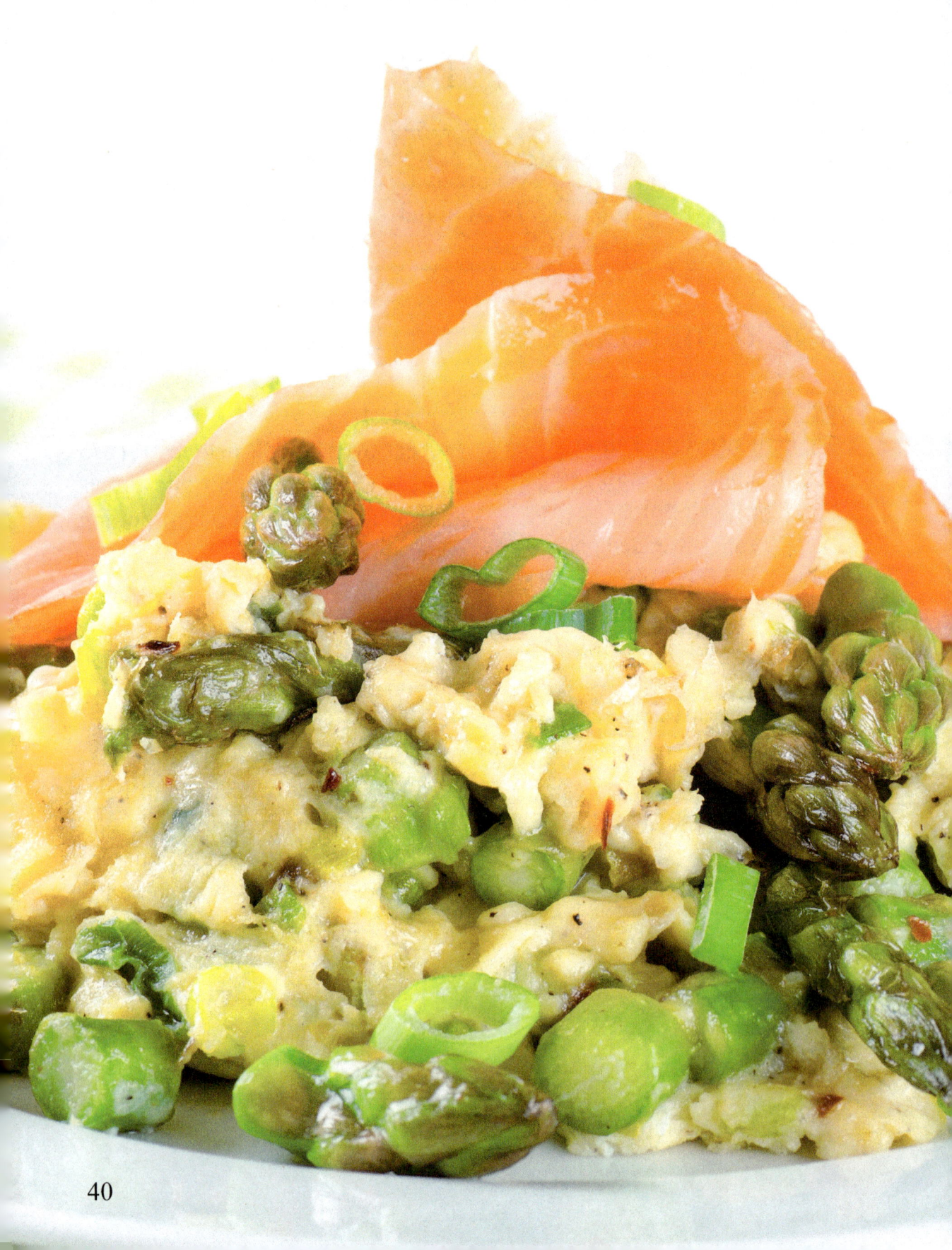

SCRAMBLED EGGS WITH ASPARAGUS & GREEN PEAS

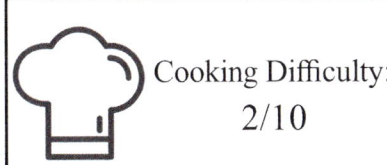 Cooking Difficulty: 2/10

 Cooking Time: 10 minutes

 Servings: 2

INGREDIENTS

- 4 eggs
- 100g green peas (frozen or fresh)
- 100g asparagus, chopped into pieces
- 100g smoked salmon, sliced
- 2 tbsp olive oil
- salt and pepper to taste
- fresh herbs for garnish (optional)

DESCRIPTION

STEP 1
Beat the eggs in a bowl, season with salt and pepper to taste. Heat olive oil in a skillet over medium heat. Add the asparagus and cook, stirring, for about 3-4 minutes until the asparagus is tender. Add the green peas to the skillet with the asparagus and cook for another 1-2 minutes.

STEP 2
Pour the beaten eggs into the skillet. Cook, stirring, until the eggs are cooked through and scrambled. Divide the scrambled eggs onto plates. Top with slices of smoked salmon and fresh herbs, if desired.

NUTRITIONAL INFORMATION
250 Calories, 15g Fat, 10g Carbs, 20g Protein

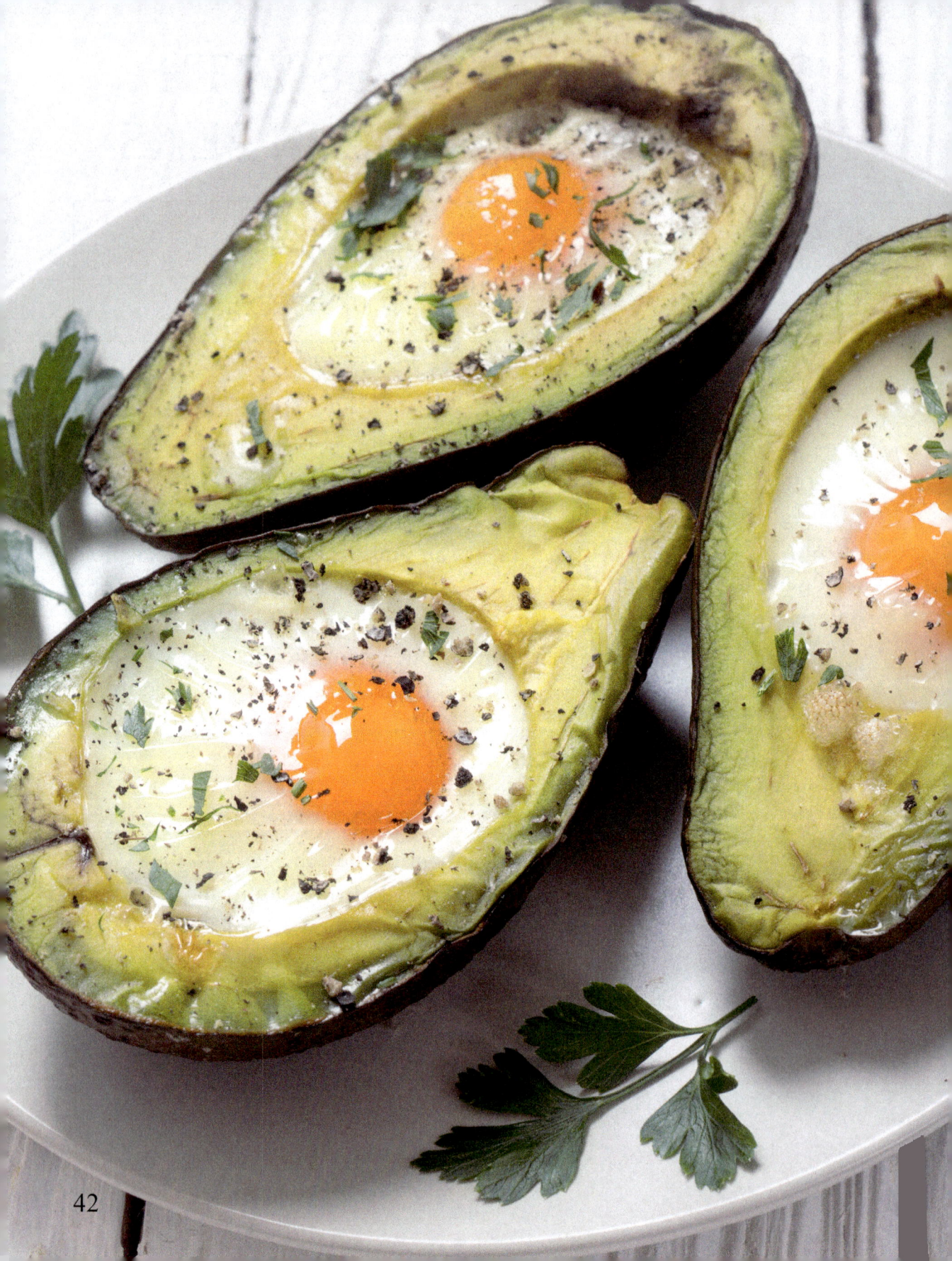

AVOCADO EGG BOATS

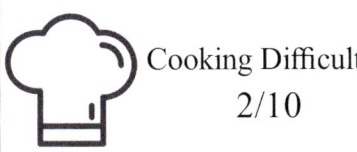 Cooking Difficulty: 2/10

 Cooking Time: 25 minutes

 Servings: 4

INGREDIENTS

- 2 ripe avocados
- 4 large eggs
- 1/4 cup chopped cilantro (for garnish)
- salt and pepper to taste

DESCRIPTION

STEP 1
Preheat oven to 350 degrees F (175 degrees C).

STEP 2
Cut avocados in half, remove the pits, and scoop out a bit of the flesh to create wells. Drizzle avocados with olive oil, salt, and pepper. Crack eggs into the avocado wells.

STEP 3
Bake for 15-20 minutes, or until egg whites are set. Garnish with cilantro before serving.

NUTRITIONAL INFORMATION

200 Calories, 3g Fat, 27g Carbs, 5g Protein

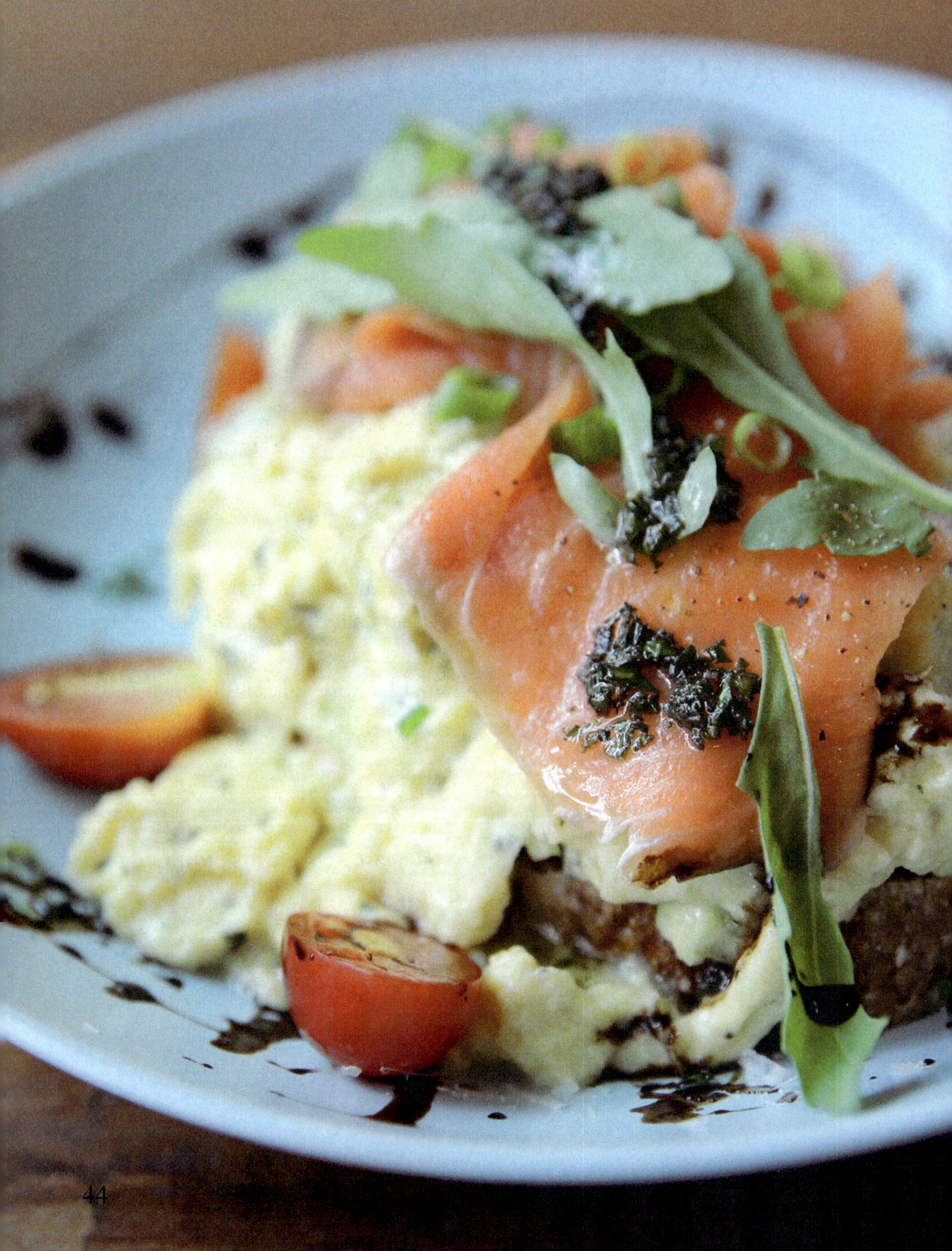

VEGETABLE AND SALMON OMELETTE

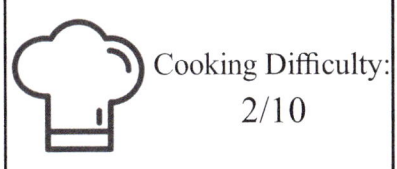 Cooking Difficulty: 2/10

 Cooking Time: 10 minutes

 Servings: 2

INGREDIENTS

- 4 eggs
- 1 small green onion, chopped
- 1 red bell pepper, chopped
- 1 small tomato, chopped
- 100g fresh salmon, diced
- 2 tbsp olive oil
- salt and pepper to taste
- fresh herbs for garnish (optional)

DESCRIPTION

STEP 1
Whisk eggs in a bowl and season with salt and pepper. Heat olive oil in a skillet over medium heat. Sauté green onion and red bell pepper for 3-4 minutes until softened. Add tomato and salmon, cook for 2-3 minutes until salmon is cooked through.

STEP 2
Pour beaten eggs into the skillet and stir gently. Cook until edges set, then lift edges with spatula and tilt skillet to allow uncooked egg to flow underneath. Once fully cooked, slide omelette onto a plate, garnish with fresh herbs if desired, and serve hot.

NUTRITIONAL INFORMATION

280 Calories, 18g Fat, 4g Carbs, 20g Protein

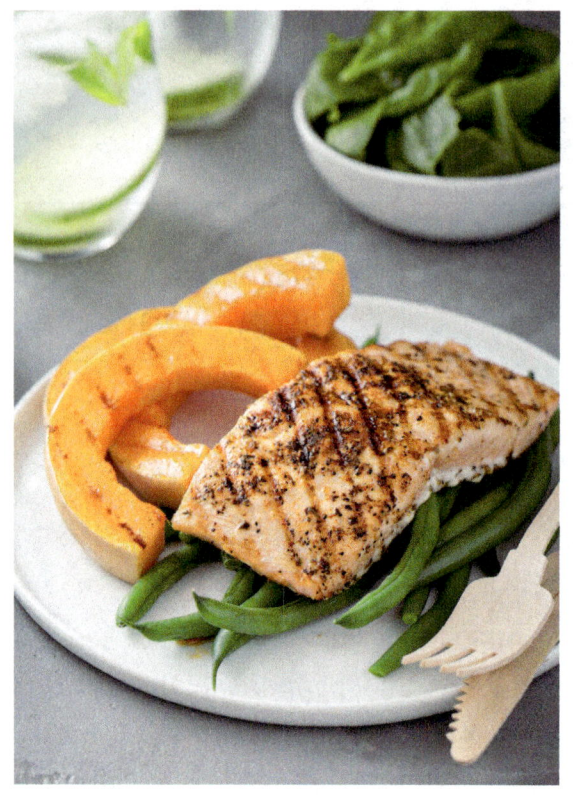
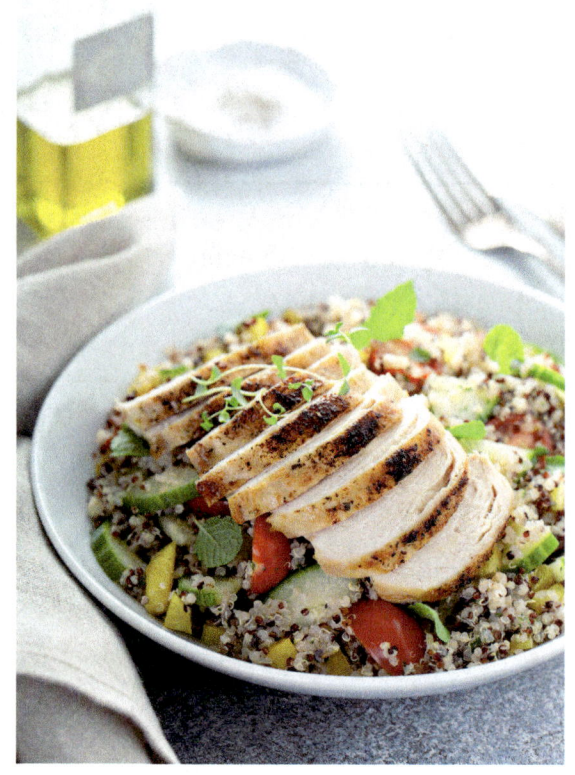
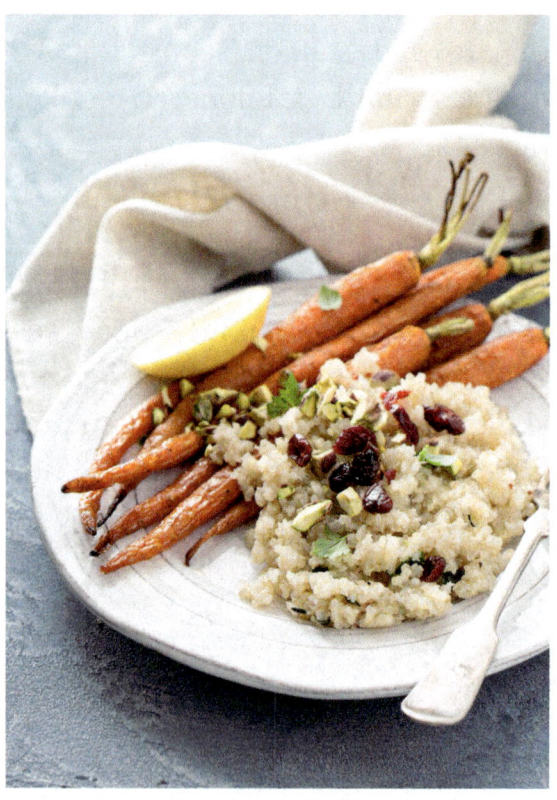
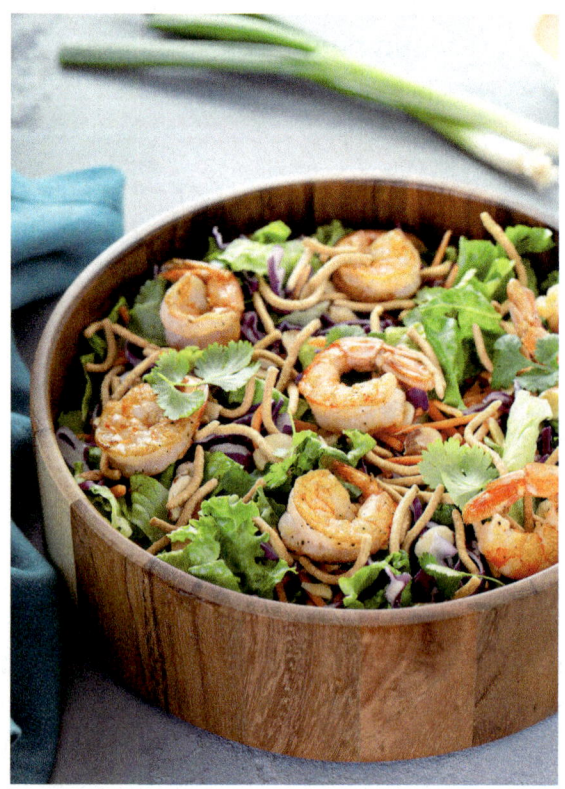

MAIN DISH

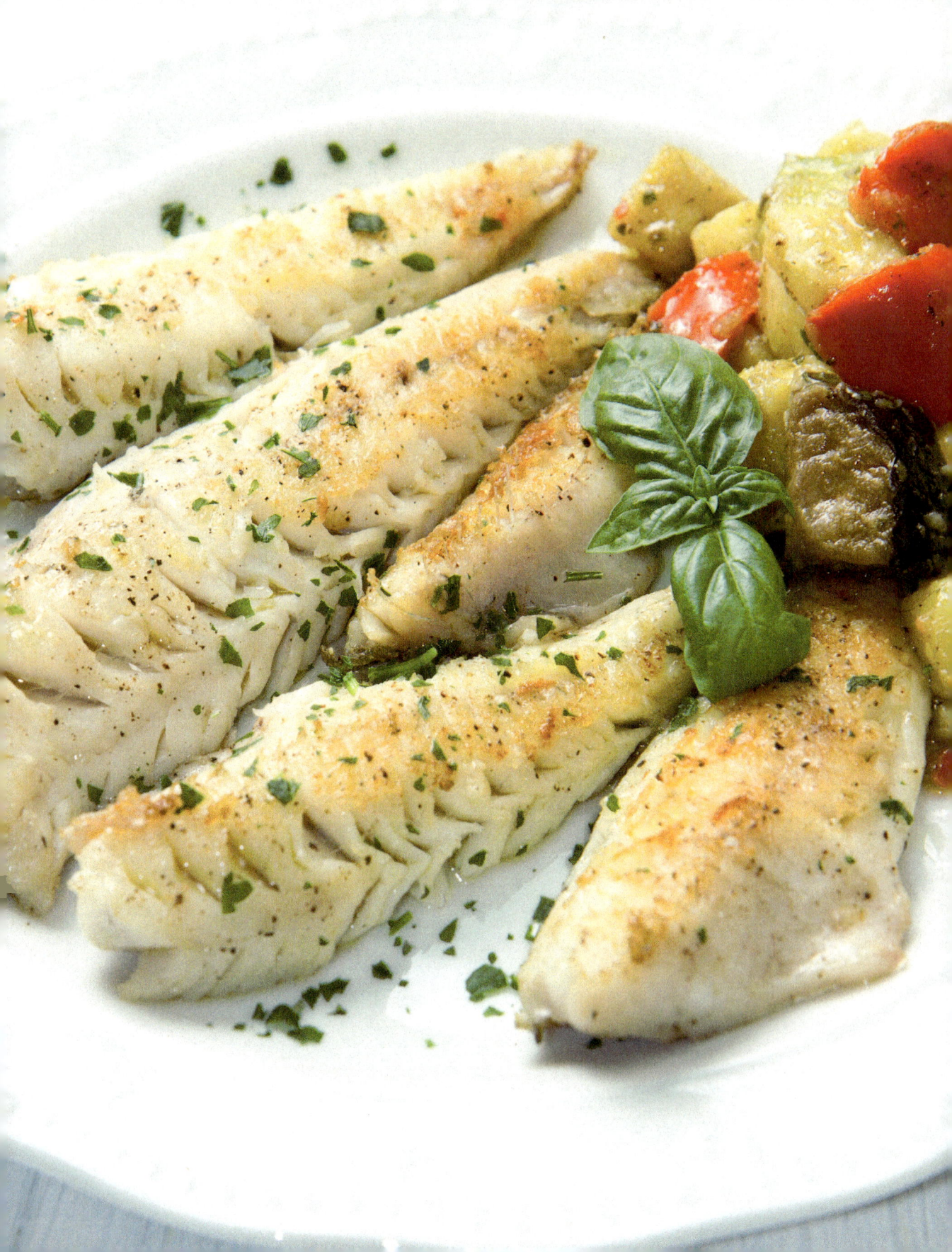

FISH WITH VEGETABLES

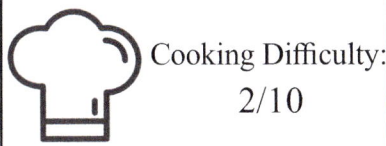 Cooking Difficulty: 2/10

 Cooking Time: 15 minutes

 Servings: 1

INGREDIENTS

- 150 grams white fish fillet (such as cod or haddock)
- 1/2 zucchini, sliced
- 1/2 bell pepper, sliced
- 1/4 red onion, sliced
- 1 tablespoon olive oil
- salt and pepper to taste

DESCRIPTION

STEP 1
Preheat the grill.

STEP 2
Cut the zucchini, bell pepper, and onion into bite-sized pieces. Drizzle the fish and vegetables with olive oil, salt, and pepper. Grill the fish for 5-7 minutes per side, or until opaque. Grill the vegetables for 3-5 minutes, or until tender.

STEP 3
Serve the fish with the grilled vegetables.

NUTRITIONAL INFORMATION

Calories: 250, Fat: 12g, Carbs: 3g, Protein: 30g

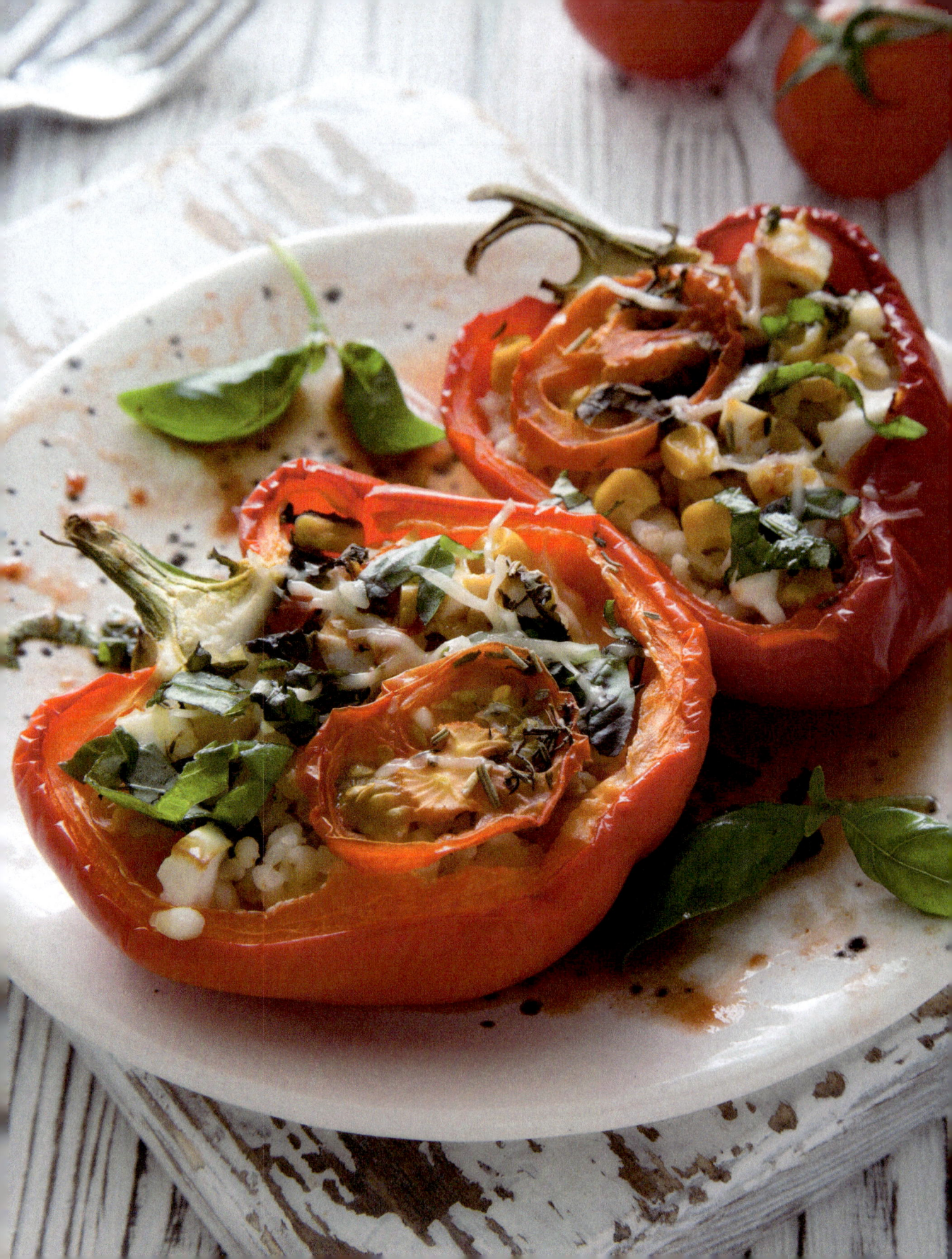

QUINOA STUFFED BELL PEPPERS

 Cooking Difficulty: 2/10

 Cooking Time: 24 minutes

 Servings: 4

INGREDIENTS

- 4 large bell peppers, halved and seeds removed
- 1 cup quinoa, cooked
- 1 can (15 oz) black beans, drained and rinsed
- 1 cup corn kernels (fresh or frozen)
- 1 cup cherry tomatoes, halved
- 1/2 cup red onion, finely chopped
- 1/2 cup fresh cilantro, chopped
- 1 teaspoon cumin
- salt and pepper to taste
- 1 cup tomato sauce (for topping)

DESCRIPTION

STEP 1
In a large mixing bowl, combine cooked quinoa, black beans, corn, cherry tomatoes, red onion, cilantro, cumin, salt, and pepper. Mix well. Stuff each bell pepper half with the quinoa mixture.

STEP 2
Preheat the air fryer at 180°C. Place the stuffed bell peppers in the air fryer basket. Cook for 15-20 minutes until the peppers are tender.

NUTRITIONAL INFORMATION

Calories 295, Fat 8 g, Carbs 11 g, Protein 9 g

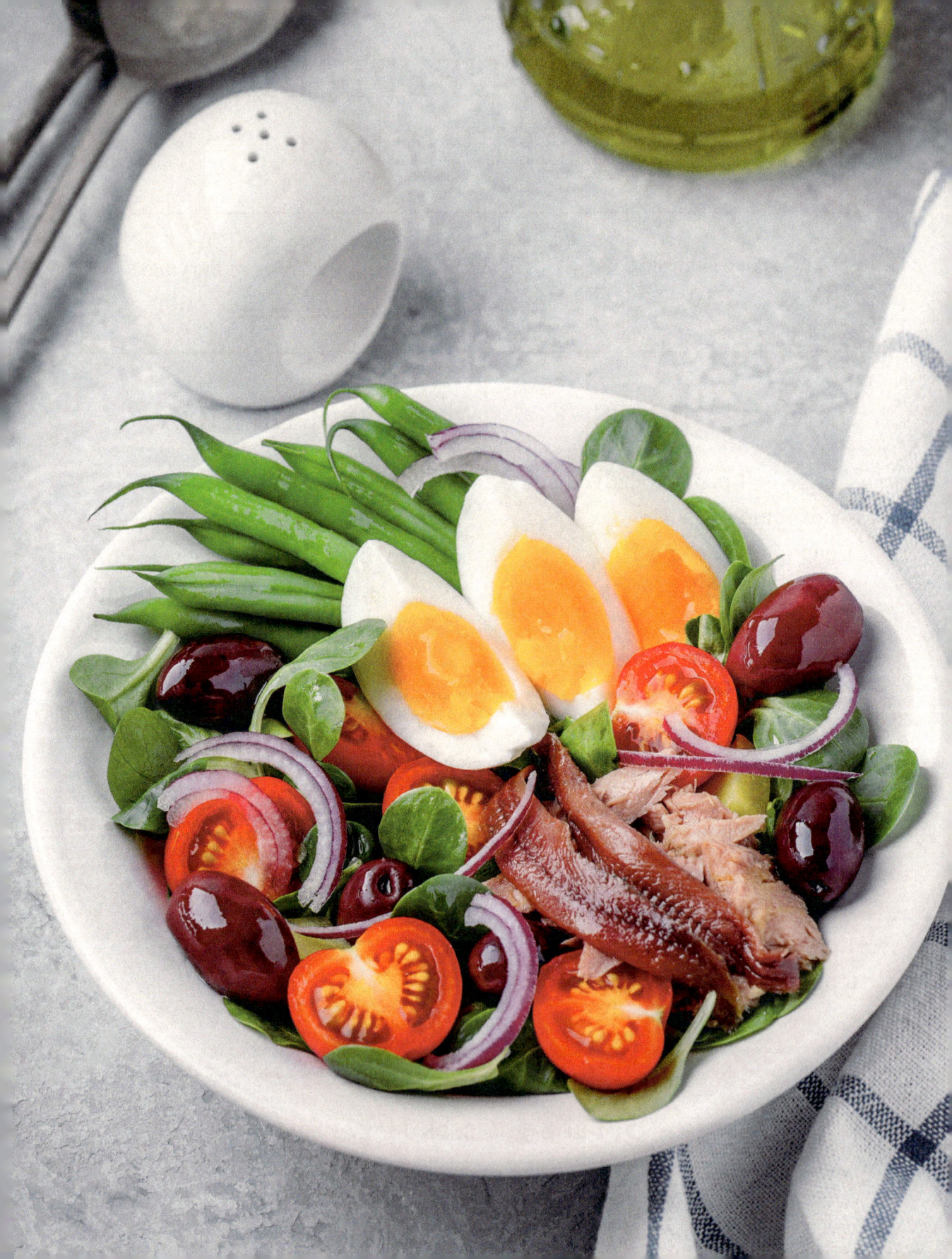

ANCHOVY SALAD WITH EGG AND CHERRY TOMATOES

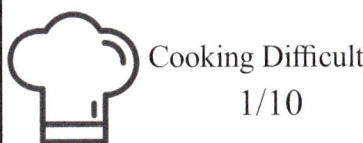 Cooking Difficulty: 1/10
 Cooking Time: 5 minutes
 Servings: 2

INGREDIENTS

- 1 oz anchovies in oil
- 1 oz kalamata olives
- 2.5 oz cherry tomatoes
- 1/4 red onion, thinly sliced
- 2.5 oz spinach
- 1 hard-boiled egg, sliced
- 1 tablespoon olive oil
- 1 tablespoon lemon juice
- salt and pepper to taste

DESCRIPTION

STEP 1
Rinse the anchovies under cold running water to remove excess salt. Chop them finely.

STEP 2
Slice the kalamata olives into rings. Halve the cherry tomatoes. In a large bowl, combine spinach, cherry tomatoes, red onion, and olives. Add the chopped anchovies and sliced egg.

STEP 3
In a small bowl, whisk together olive oil, lemon juice, salt, and pepper. Dress the salad with the prepared mixture and toss gently.

NUTRITIONAL INFORMATION

Calories: 280, Fat: 8g, Carbs: 8g, Protein: 4g

CHICKEN CHICKPEA SOUP WITH VEGETABLES

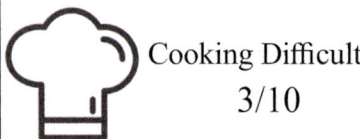 Cooking Difficulty: 3/10	 Cooking Time: 45 minutes	 Servings: 2

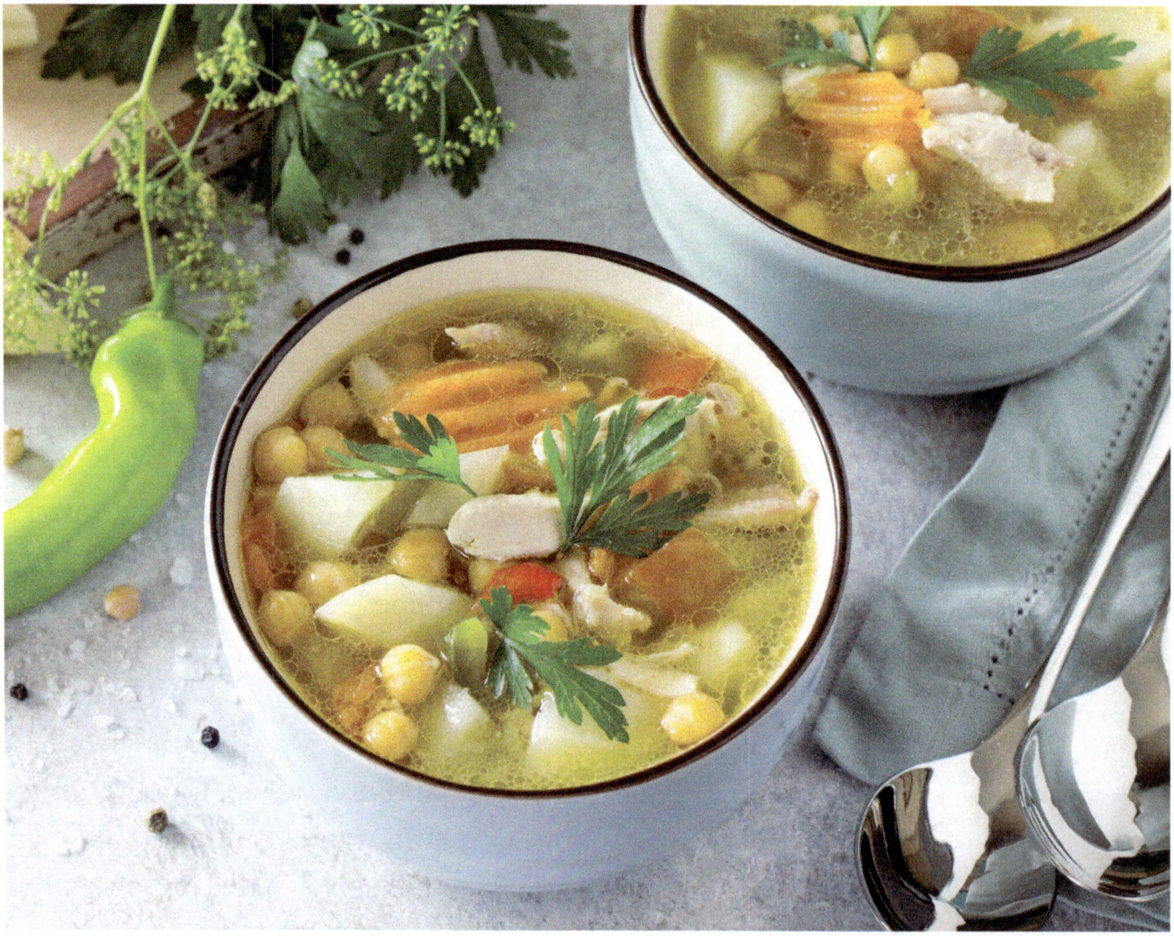

NUTRITIONAL INFORMATION

Calories 360, Fat 18g, Carbs 15g, Protein 30g

INGREDIENTS

- 1 boneless, skinless chicken breast (about 5 oz)
- 1/2 cup dried chickpeas, soaked overnight
- 1 onion, chopped
- 1 carrot, chopped
- 1 celery stalk, chopped
- 2 garlic cloves, minced
- 1 tomato, diced
- 4 cups chicken broth
- 1 bay leaf
- 1/2 teaspoon dried thyme
- salt and pepper to taste
- fresh parsley for garnish (optional)

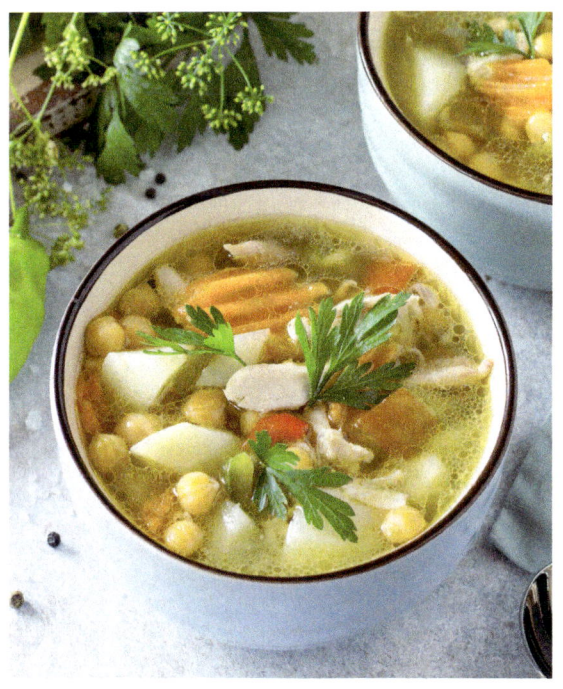

DESCRIPTION

STEP 1
Cook the chicken in a pot of boiling water until cooked through, about 15-20 minutes. Remove from pot, cool, and shred. Strain the broth.

STEP 2
Sauté the onion, carrot, and celery in olive oil until softened, about 5-7 minutes. Add the garlic, tomato, bay leaf, and thyme and cook for 2 more minutes.

STEP 3
Drain the chickpeas and add them to the pot. Pour in the chicken broth and bring to a boil. Reduce heat and simmer for 20-25 minutes, or until the chickpeas are tender.

STEP 4
Season with salt and pepper to taste.

STEP 5
Serve the soup with the shredded chicken and garnish with parsley, if desired.

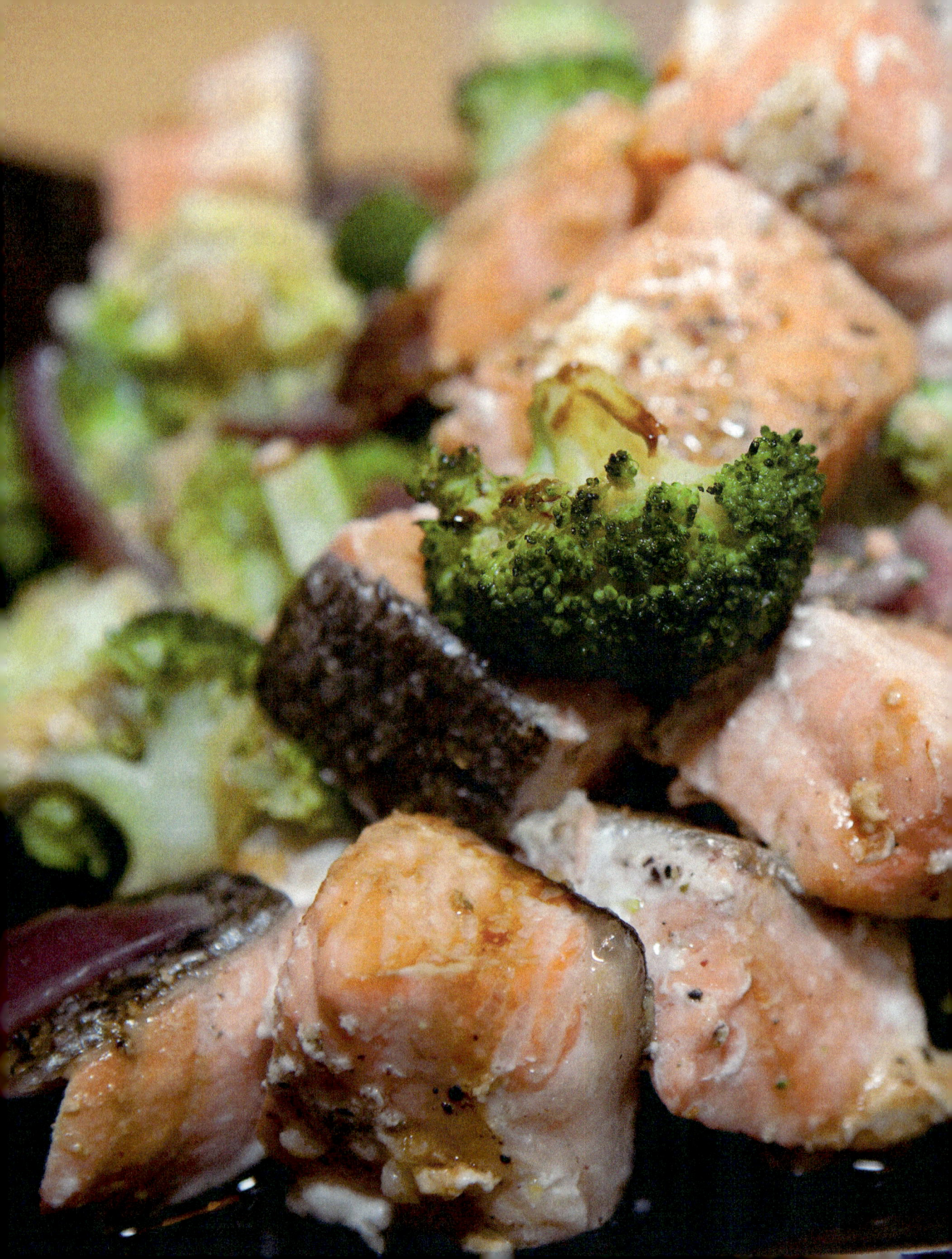

SALMON WITH BROCCOLI

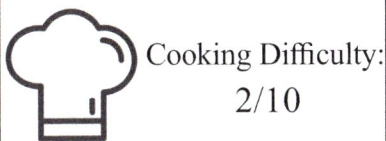 Cooking Difficulty: 2/10

 Cooking Time: 22 minutes

 Servings: 2

INGREDIENTS

- 7 oz (200 g) salmon fillet, cut into cubes
- 5 oz (150 g) broccoli florets
- ¼ red onion, diced
- 1 tablespoon olive oil
- ½ teaspoon salt
- ¼ teaspoon black pepper
- 1 tablespoon lemon juice (optional)

DESCRIPTION

STEP 1
Preheat oven to 400°F (200°C).

STEP 2
In a bowl, combine salmon, broccoli, red onion, olive oil, salt, and pepper. Spread mixture on a baking sheet lined with parchment paper. Bake for 15-20 minutes, or until salmon is opaque and broccoli is tender.

STEP 3
Drizzle with lemon juice before serving, if desired.

NUTRITIONAL INFORMATION

400 Calories, 25g Fat, 5g Carbs, 35g Protein

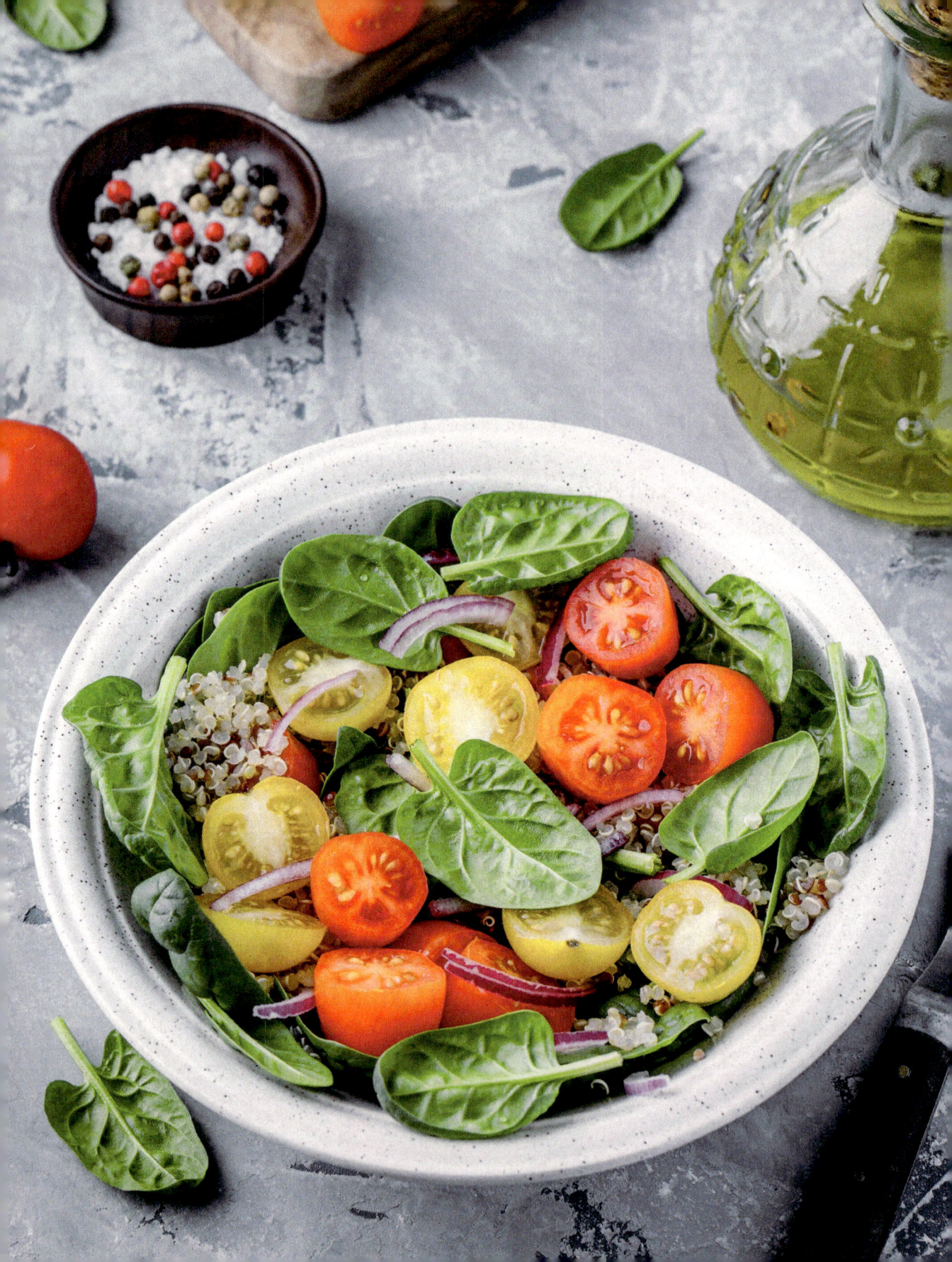

FRESH QUINOA SALAD

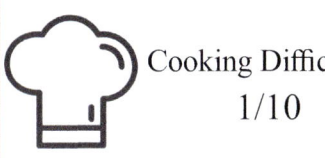 Cooking Difficulty: 1/10

 Cooking Time: 18 minutes

 Servings: 2

INGREDIENTS

- 1/2 cup (100 g) quinoa, rinsed
- 1 cup (240 ml) water or vegetable broth
- 1 cup (50 g) baby spinach
- 1 cup (150 g) cherry tomatoes, halved
- 1/4 cup (30 g) red onion, thinly sliced
- 2 tablespoons olive oil
- 1 tablespoon lemon juice
- salt and freshly ground black pepper to taste

DESCRIPTION

STEP 1
Cook quinoa according to package instructions (about 15 minutes). Let cool slightly.

STEP 2
Combine quinoa, spinach, tomatoes, and red onion in a large bowl. In a small bowl, whisk together olive oil, lemon juice, salt, and pepper.

STEP 3
Pour the dressing over the salad and toss to coat. Serve immediately or refrigerate for up to 2 days.

NUTRITIONAL INFORMATION

Calories: 250, Fat: 5g, Carbs: 7g, Protein: 11g

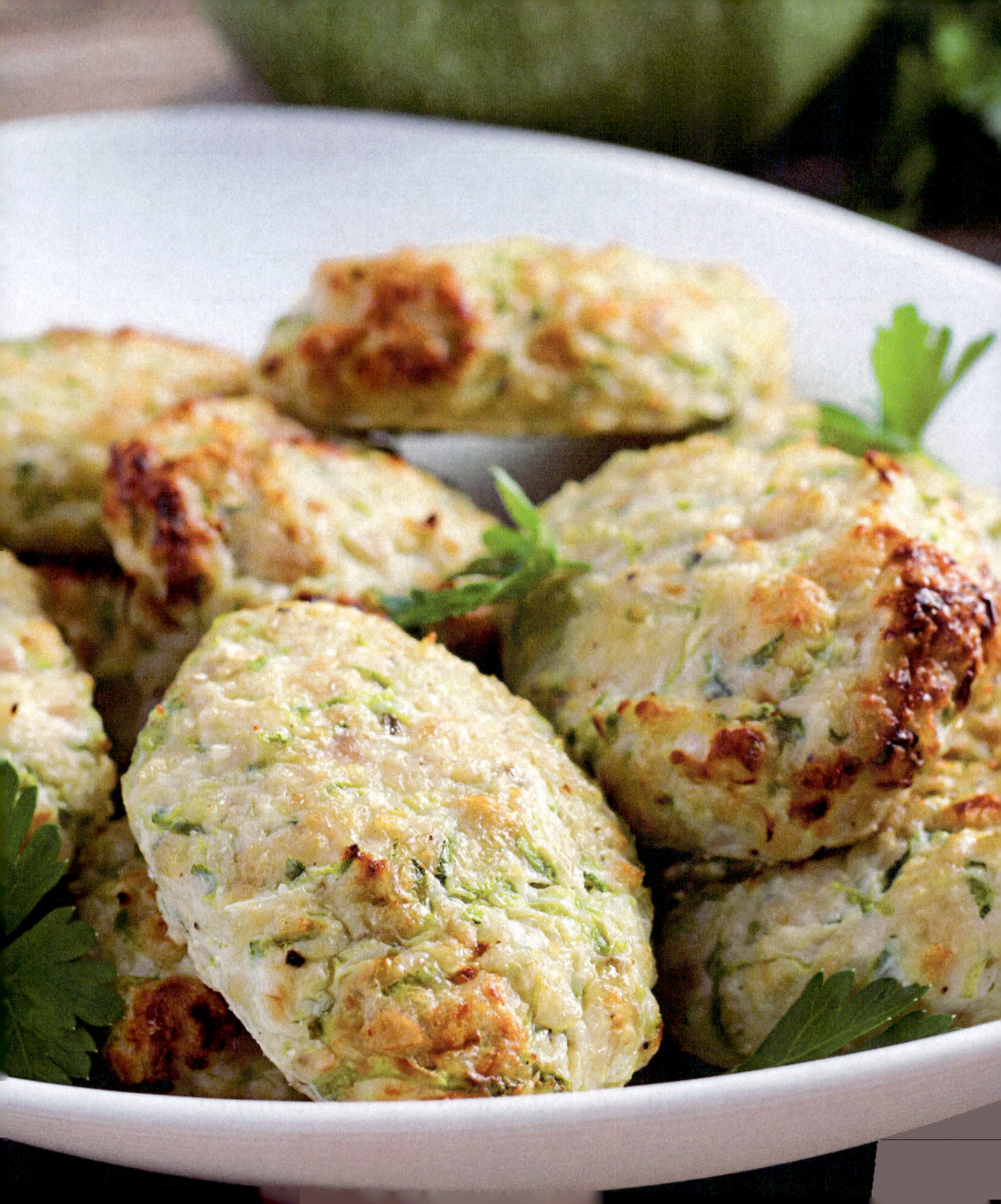

CHICKEN MEATBALLS WITH ZUCCHINI

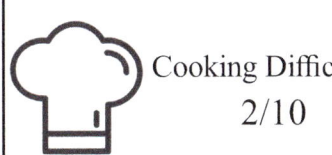 Cooking Difficulty: 2/10

 Cooking Time: 28 minutes

 Servings: 4

INGREDIENTS

- 1 pound ground chicken
- 1 zucchini, grated
- 1/2 onion, finely chopped
- 1 clove garlic, finely chopped
- 1/2 cup rolled oats
- 1 tablespoon olive oil
- 1 teaspoon salt
- 1/2 teaspoon black pepper
- 1/4 teaspoon oregano
- 1/4 teaspoon basil

DESCRIPTION

STEP 1
Preheat the oven to 400°F (200°C). Line a baking sheet with parchment paper or lightly grease it.

STEP 2
In a large bowl, combine chicken, zucchini, onion, garlic, oats, olive oil, salt, pepper, oregano, and basil.

STEP 3
Shape the chicken mixture into meatballs and place them on the prepared baking sheet. Bake in the oven for 20-25 minutes, flipping the meatballs halfway through, until golden brown and cooked through.

NUTRITIONAL INFORMATION

Calories: 230, Fat: 10g, Carbs: 15g, Protein: 20g

SALMON WITH SPINACH

 Cooking Difficulty: 1/10

 Cooking Time: 15 minutes

 Servings: 2

INGREDIENTS

- 2 salmon fillets
- 1 tablespoon olive oil
- 1 garlic clove, minced
- juice of 1/2 lemon
- salt and pepper, to taste
- 2 cups fresh spinach

DESCRIPTION

STEP 1
Preheat the oven to 400°F (200°C). Place salmon on a baking sheet lined with parchment. Add all remaining ingredients except for the spinach. Bake for 12-15 minutes. In a skillet, add a small amount of olive oil and sauté spinach until wilted, about 2-3 minutes. Serve and enjoy!

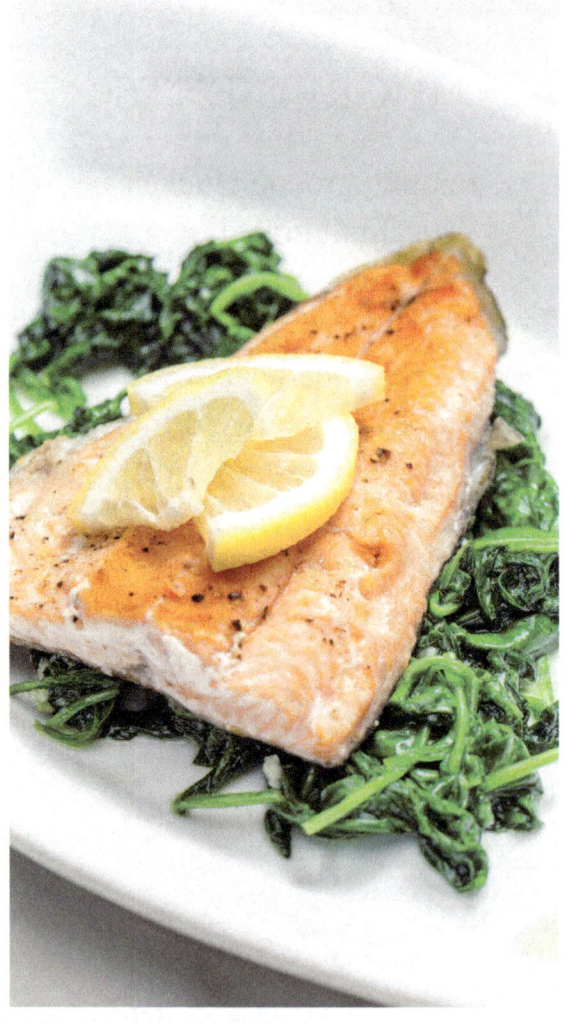

NUTRITIONAL INFORMATION

310 Calories, 11g Fat, 15g Carbs, 15g Protein

SPINACH AND BERRY SALAD

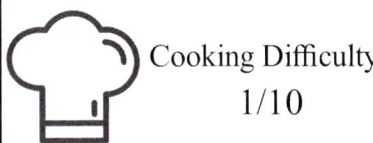 Cooking Difficulty: 1/10

 Cooking Time: 4 minutes

 Servings: 2

INGREDIENTS

- 2 cups fresh spinach
- 1/2 cup mixed berries (strawberries, blueberries, or raspberries)
- 2 tablespoons walnuts or almonds, chopped
- 1 tablespoon olive oil
- 1 teaspoon balsamic vinegar
- salt and pepper, to taste

DESCRIPTION

STEP 1
In a bowl, combine spinach, berries, and nuts. Drizzle with olive oil and balsamic vinegar, season with salt and pepper, and toss to combine. Enjoy immediately.

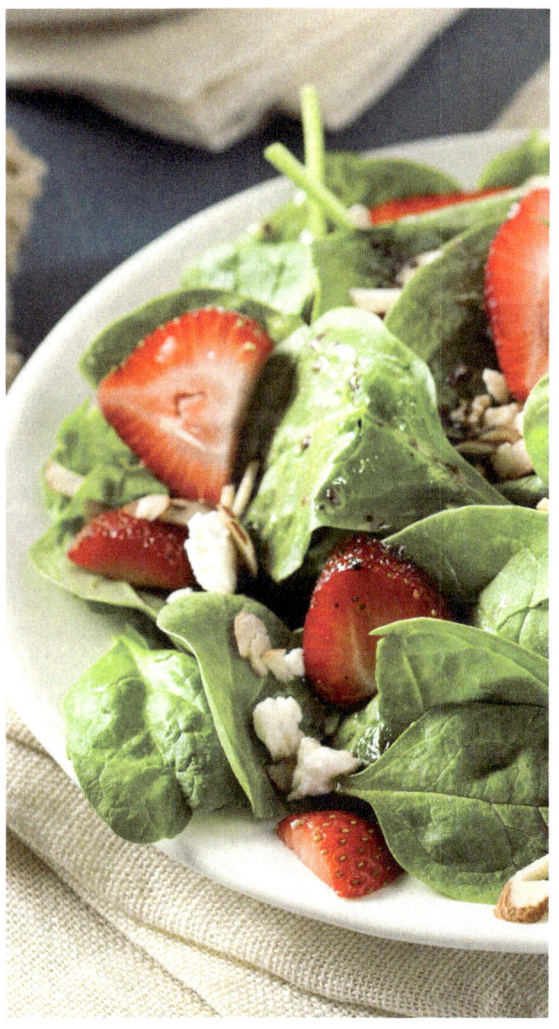

NUTRITIONAL INFORMATION

100 Calories, 5g Fat, 3g Carbs, 1g Protein

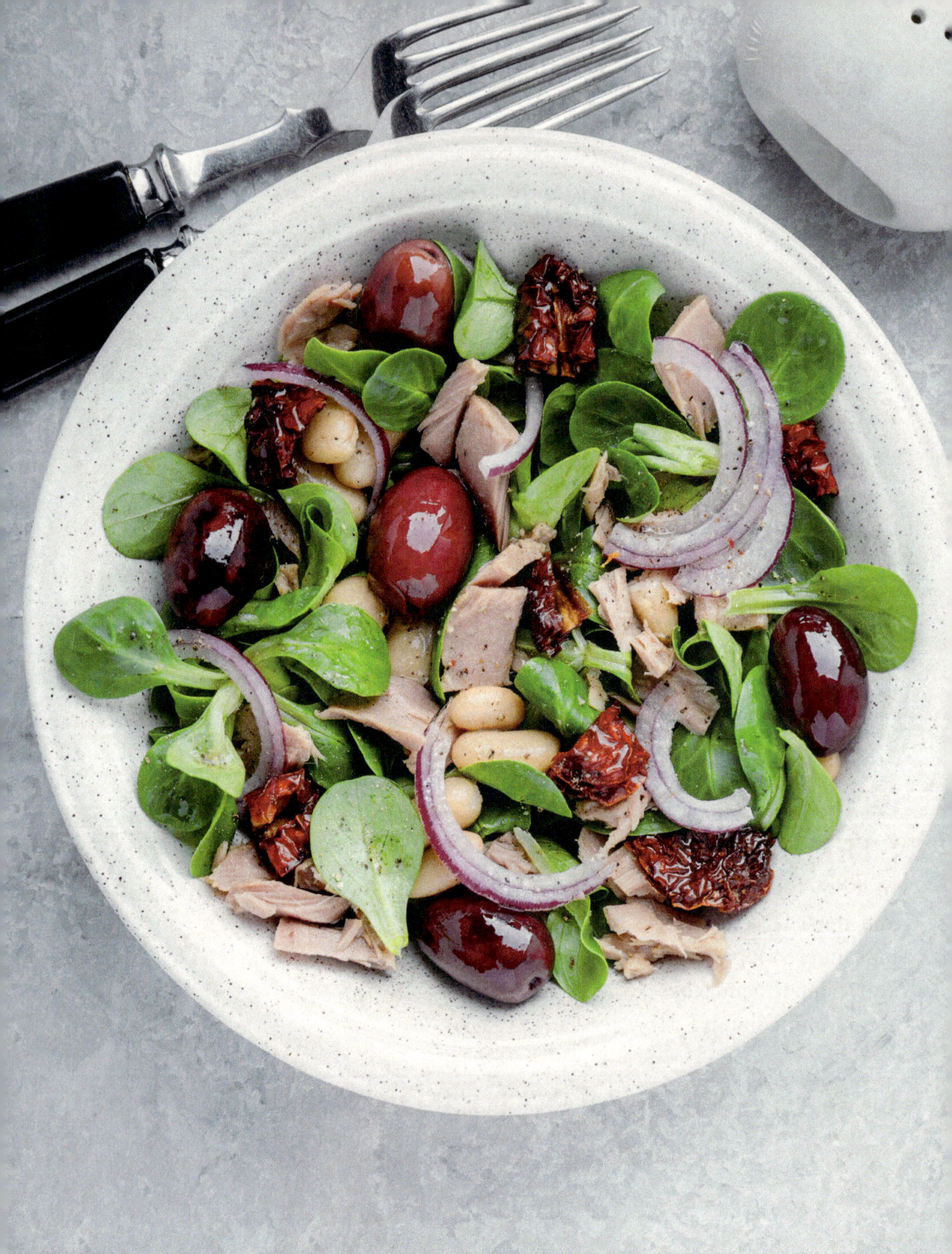

TUNA SALAD WITH SPINACH

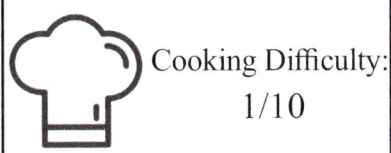 Cooking Difficulty: 1/10

 Cooking Time: 2 minutes

 Servings: 2

INGREDIENTS

- 1 (5-ounce) can tuna in olive oil, drained and flaked
- 4 cups baby spinach
- 1/2 cup sun-dried tomatoes, sliced
- 1/2 cup cooked white beans, drained and rinsed
- 1/4 cup whole olives, pitted
- 1/4 cup red onion, thinly sliced
- 2 tablespoons olive oil
- 1 tablespoon lemon juice
- 1/2 teaspoon salt
- 1/4 teaspoon black pepper

DESCRIPTION

STEP 1
In a large bowl, combine the tuna, spinach, sun-dried tomatoes, white beans, olives, and red onion.

STEP 2
In a small bowl, whisk together the olive oil, lemon juice, salt, and pepper.

STEP 3
Pour the dressing over the salad and toss to coat. Serve immediately.

NUTRITIONAL INFORMATION

Calories: 350, Fat: 15g, Carbs: 30g, Protein: 25g

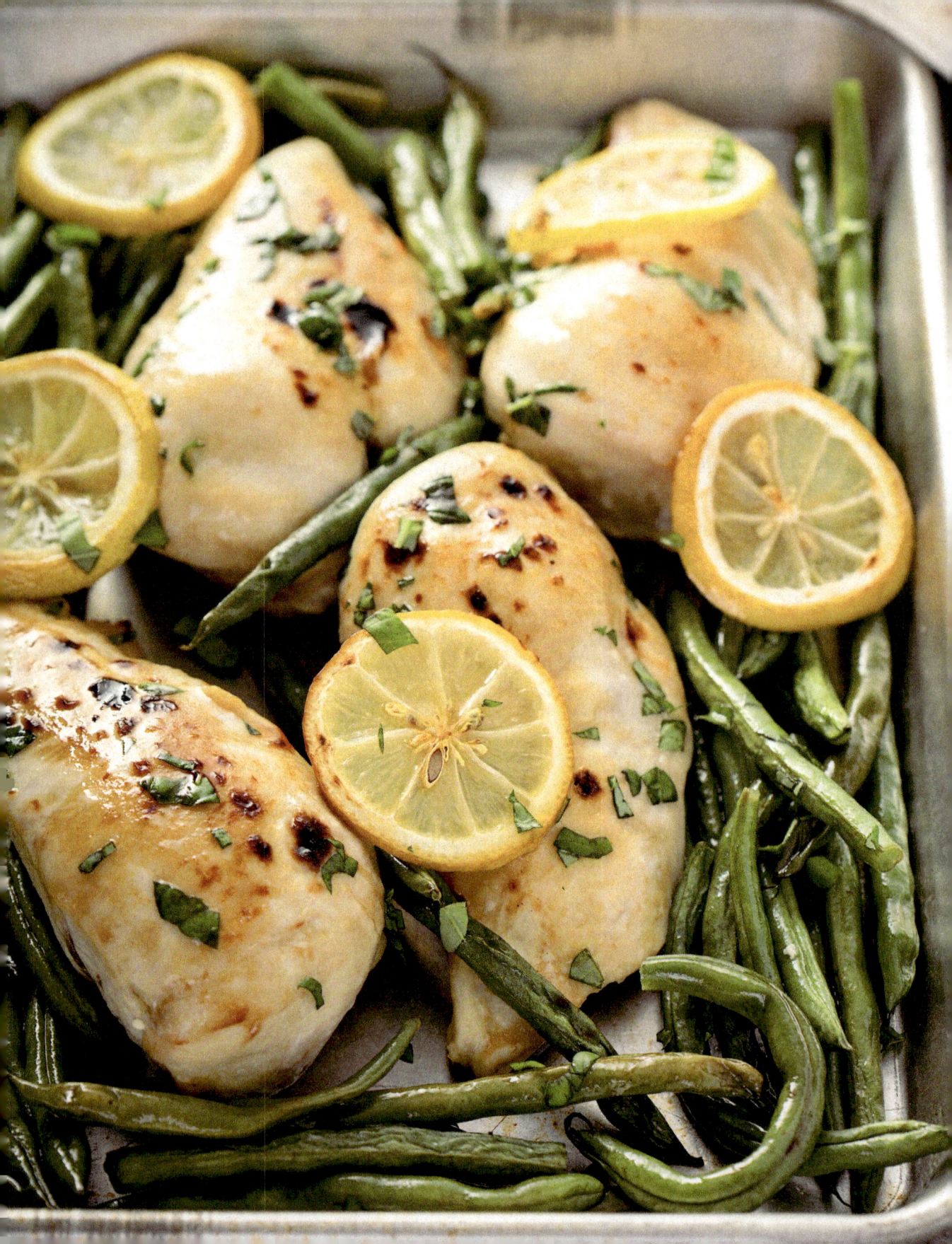

LEMON HERB BAKED CHICKEN

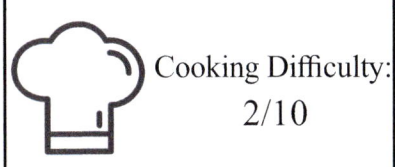 Cooking Difficulty: 2/10

 Cooking Time: 57 minutes

 Servings: 4

INGREDIENTS

- 4 boneless, skinless chicken breasts (about 3 lbs)
- 2 tablespoons olive oil
- 1 tablespoon lemon juice
- 1 teaspoon dried oregano
- 1/2 teaspoon dried thyme
- 1/4 teaspoon garlic powder
- 1/4 teaspoon paprika
- salt and freshly ground black pepper to taste
- 1 pound (450 g) green beans, trimmed and cut into bite-sized pieces
- 1 lemon, thinly sliced

DESCRIPTION

STEP 1
Preheat your oven to 400°F (200°C). In a small bowl, whisk together olive oil, lemon juice, oregano, thyme, garlic powder, paprika, salt, and pepper.

STEP 2
Place chicken breasts in a baking dish. Pour the marinade over the chicken, ensuring they're evenly coated. Arrange the green beans around the chicken breasts. Top with lemon slices.

STEP 3
Bake for 30-35 minutes, or until the chicken is cooked through. Let the chicken rest for a few minutes before serving.

NUTRITIONAL INFORMATION

Calories: 300, Fat: 12g, Carbs: 15g, Protein: 35g

SHRIMP POWER BOWL

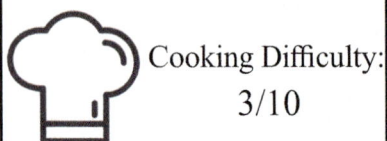 Cooking Difficulty: 3/10

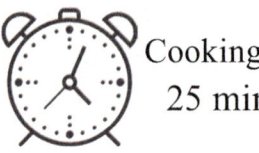 Cooking Time: 25 minutes

 Servings: 2

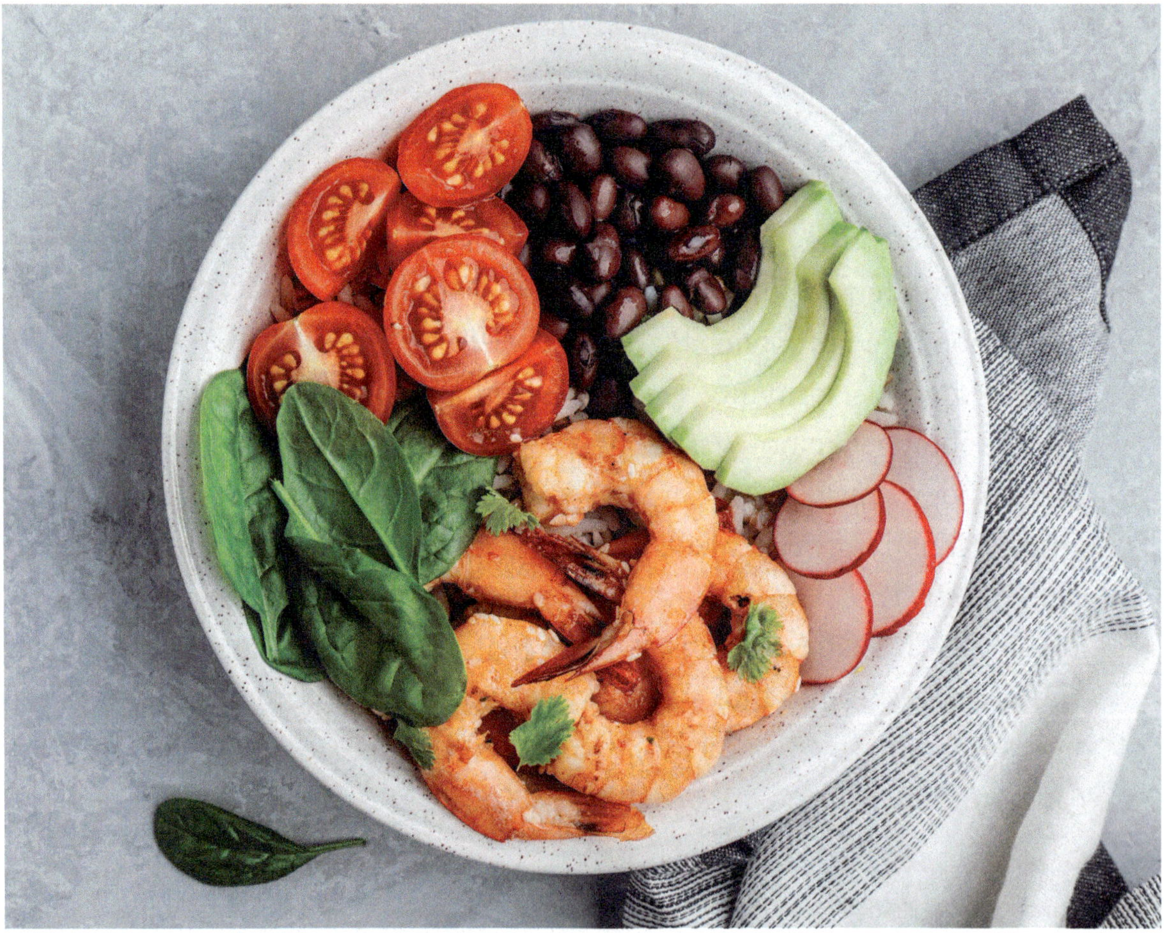

NUTRITIONAL INFORMATION

Calories 450, Fat 18g, Carbs 45g, Protein 30g

INGREDIENTS

for the rice:
- 1/2 cup (100 g) brown rice or quinoa, cooked according to package directions

for the shrimp:
- 1 pound (450 g) shrimp, peeled and deveined
- 1 tablespoon olive oil
- 1/2 teaspoon garlic powder
- 1/4 teaspoon salt
- 1/4 teaspoon black pepper

for the toppings:
- 1 can (15 ounces) red kidney beans, drained and rinsed
- 1 avocado, sliced
- 5 radishes, thinly sliced
- 10 cherry tomatoes, halved
- 2 tablespoons chopped cilantro

for the dressing:
- 1/4 cup olive oil
- 2 tablespoons lime juice
- 1 tablespoon honey
- 1 teaspoon dijon mustard
- 1/2 teaspoon salt
- 1/4 teaspoon black pepper

DESCRIPTION

STEP 1
Cook the rice or quinoa according to package directions.

STEP 2
In a medium bowl, combine the shrimp, olive oil, garlic powder, salt, and pepper. Let marinate for 5 minutes.

STEP 3
Heat a large skillet over medium-high heat. Add the shrimp and cook until pink and cooked through, about 2-3 minutes per side.

STEP 4
Divide the rice or quinoa evenly among two bowls. Top with the shrimp, red kidney beans, avocado, radishes, cherry tomatoes, and cilantro.

STEP 5
In a small bowl, whisk together the olive oil, lime juice, honey, Dijon mustard, salt, and pepper. Drizzle the dressing over the bowls and serve immediately.

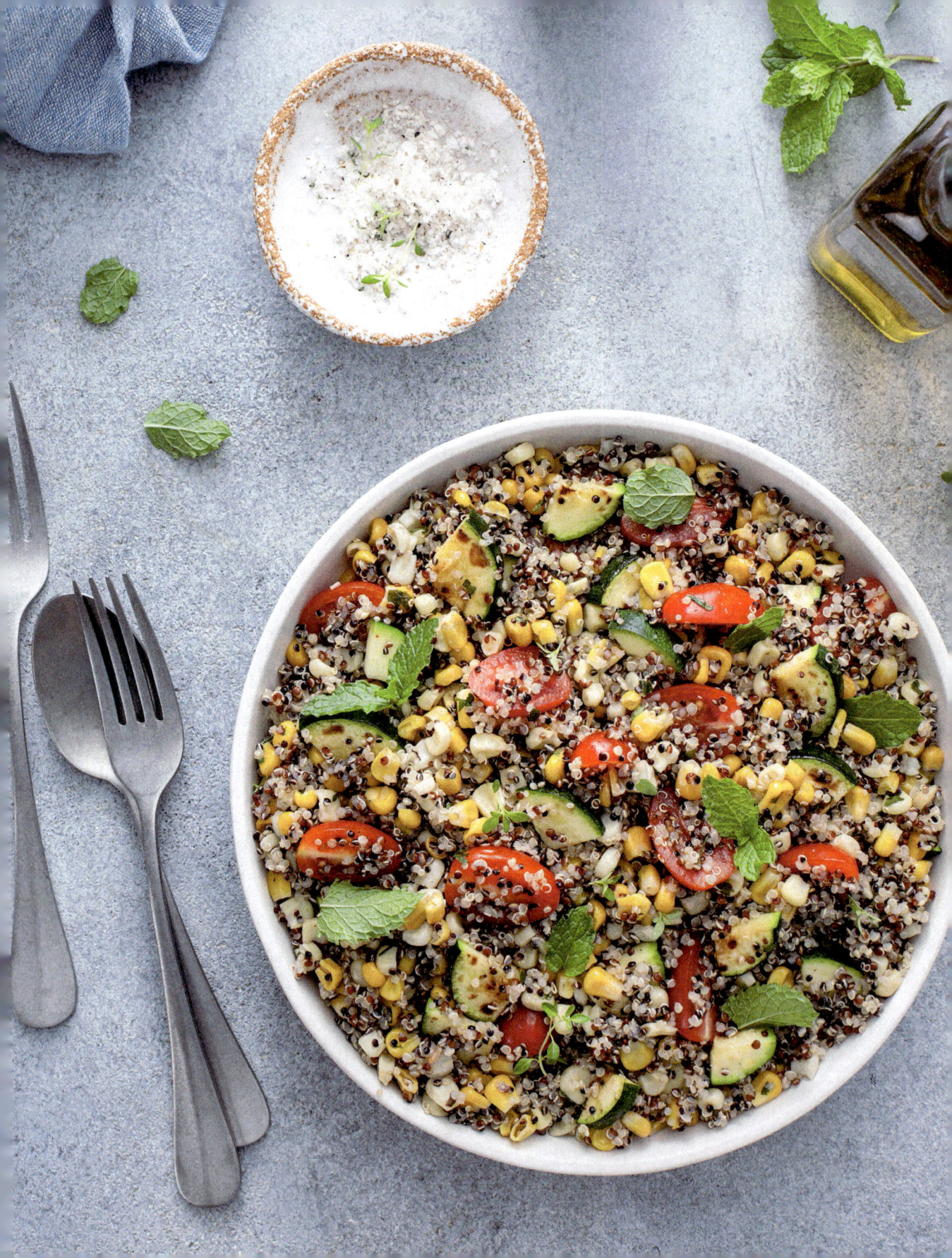

SUMMER QUINOA SALAD

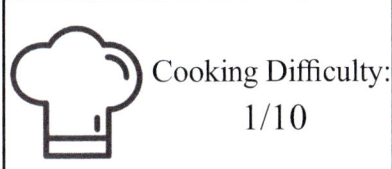 Cooking Difficulty: 1/10

 Cooking Time: 18 minutes

 Servings: 2

INGREDIENTS

for the salad:
- 1/2 cup (100 g) quinoa, rinsed
- 1 cup (240 ml) water or vegetable broth
- 1 cup (150 g) cherry tomatoes, halved
- 1 small zucchini, diced
- 1/2 cup (75 g) frozen corn kernels, thawed (or 1/2 cup fresh corn kernels)
- 1/4 cup (chopped fresh parsley or cilantro)

for the dressing:
- 2 tablespoons olive oil
- 1 tablespoon lemon juice
- 1/2 teaspoon dijon mustard
- salt and freshly ground black pepper to taste

DESCRIPTION

STEP 1
In a saucepan, combine the quinoa and water or broth. Bring to a boil, then reduce heat, cover, and simmer for 15 minutes, or until the quinoa is cooked through and fluffy.

STEP 2
While the quinoa cools, halve the cherry tomatoes, dice the zucchini, and fresh corn kernels. Chop the parsley or cilantro.

STEP 3
In a small bowl, whisk together the olive oil, lemon juice, Dijon mustard, salt, and pepper. Pour the dressing over the salad and toss gently to coat.

NUTRITIONAL INFORMATION

Calories: 250, Fat: 5g, Carbs: 7g, Protein: 11g

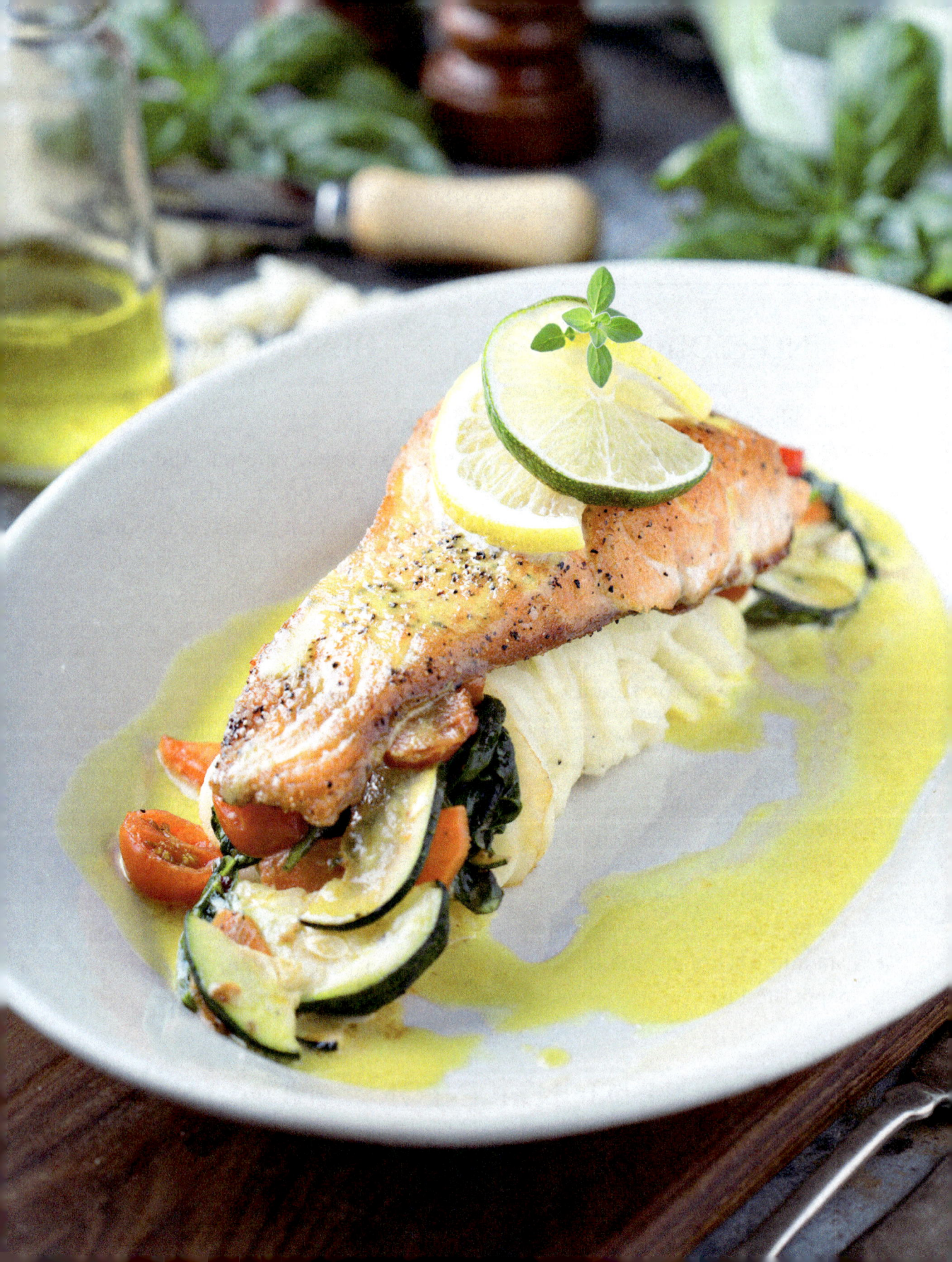

BAKED SALMON WITH LEMON AND HERBS

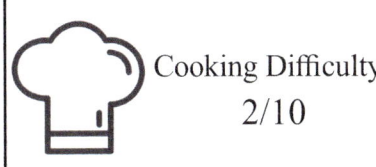 Cooking Difficulty: 2/10

 Cooking Time: 25 minutes

 Servings: 2

INGREDIENTS

- 2 salmon fillets (about 6 ounces each)
- 1 tablespoon olive oil
- 1/2 teaspoon salt
- 1/4 teaspoon black pepper
- 1/4 teaspoon dried oregano
- 1/4 teaspoon dried thyme
- 1 lemon, thinly sliced (optional)

DESCRIPTION

STEP 1
Preheat oven to 400 degrees F (200 degrees C). Line a baking sheet with parchment paper.

STEP 2
In a small bowl, combine olive oil, salt, pepper, oregano, and thyme. Place salmon fillets on the prepared baking sheet and spread the spice mixture evenly over them. Top with lemon slices, if using.

STEP 3
Bake for 15-20 minutes, or until salmon is cooked through. Serve baked salmon with your favorite vegetables.

NUTRITIONAL INFORMATION

Calories: 230, Fat: 10g, Carbs: 10g, Protein: 12g

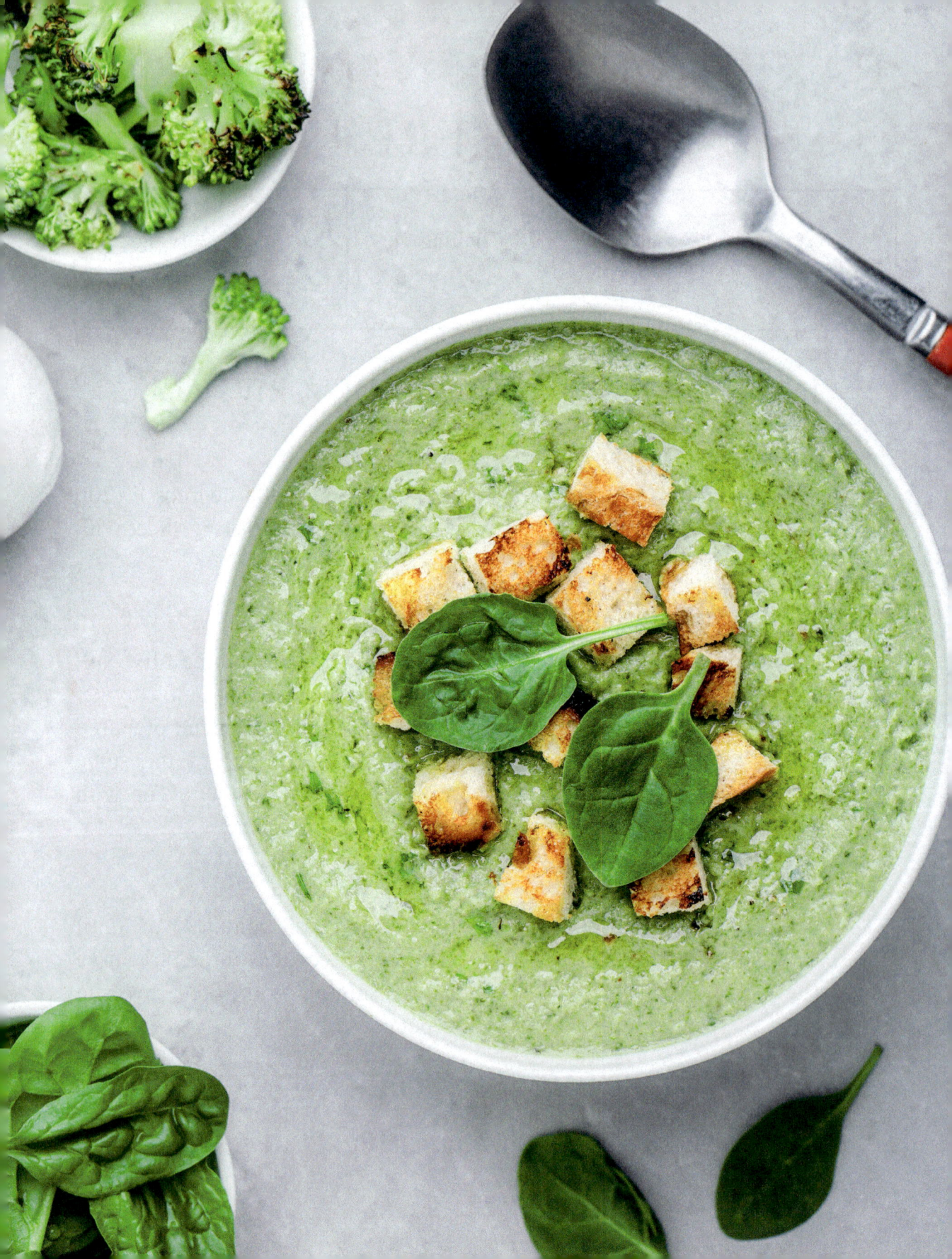

SPINACH AND BROCCOLI SOUP

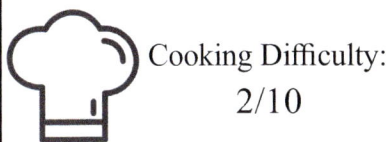 Cooking Difficulty: 2/10

 Cooking Time: 27 minutes

 Servings: 2

INGREDIENTS

- 1 tablespoon olive oil
- 1 onion, diced
- 2 cloves garlic, minced
- 1 cup broccoli florets
- 1 cup frozen spinach
- 3 cups vegetable broth
- ⅓ cup unsweetened coconut milk (optional)
- salt and pepper to taste

DESCRIPTION

STEP 1
Sauté onion and garlic, add broccoli and spinach, cook until softened.

STEP 2
Pour in vegetable broth, bring to a boil, simmer 15 minutes.

STEP 3
Blend until smooth, add coconut milk (optional), salt, and pepper.

STEP 4
Heat through, serve hot.

NUTRITIONAL INFORMATION

Calories: 200, Fat: 10g, Carbs: 10g, Protein: 5g

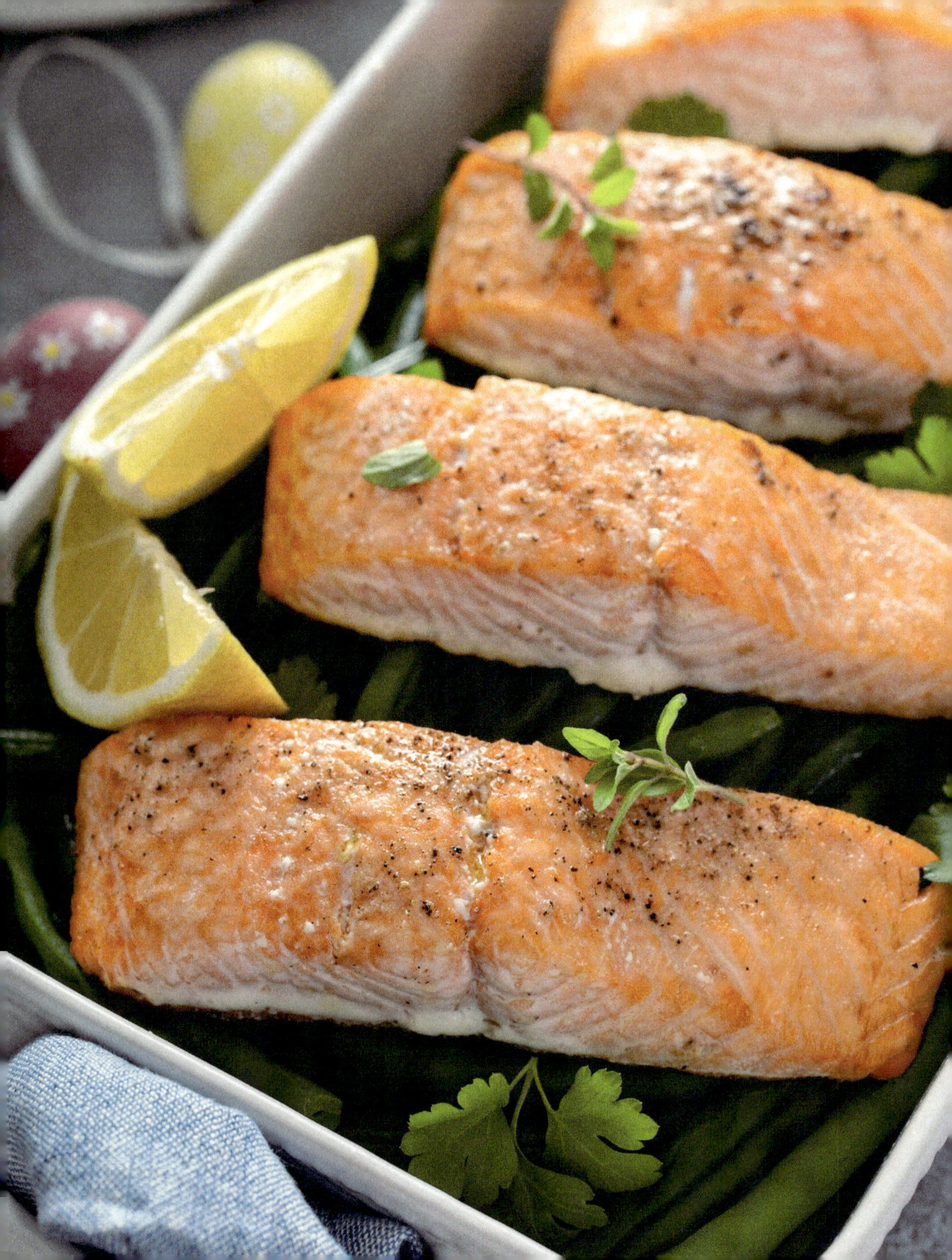

BAKED SALMON WITH GREEN BEANS

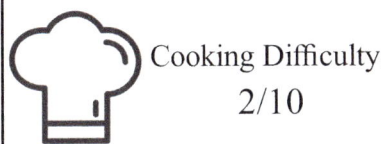 Cooking Difficulty: 2/10

 Cooking Time: 25 minutes

 Servings: 4

INGREDIENTS

- 4 salmon fillets (about 5.5 ounces each)
- 14 ounces green beans, trimmed
- 1 tablespoon olive oil
- 1/2 teaspoon salt
- 1/4 teaspoon black pepper
- 1 lemon, sliced
- 1/4 cup fresh parsley, chopped

DESCRIPTION

STEP 1
Preheat oven to 400 degrees F (200 degrees C). Wash and trim the green beans. Blanch in boiling water for 2-3 minutes, then drain and set aside. In a large bowl, toss the green beans with olive oil, salt, and pepper.

STEP 2
Spread the green beans in a baking dish. Place the salmon fillets on top of the green beans. Season the salmon with salt, pepper, and lemon slices. Bake for 15-20 minutes, or until the salmon is cooked through. Garnish with parsley and serve.

NUTRITIONAL INFORMATION

Calories: 400, Fat: 18g, Carbs: 10g, Protein: 30g

EGGPLANT MELANGE

 Cooking Difficulty: 3/10	 Cooking Time: 34 minutes	 Servings: 2

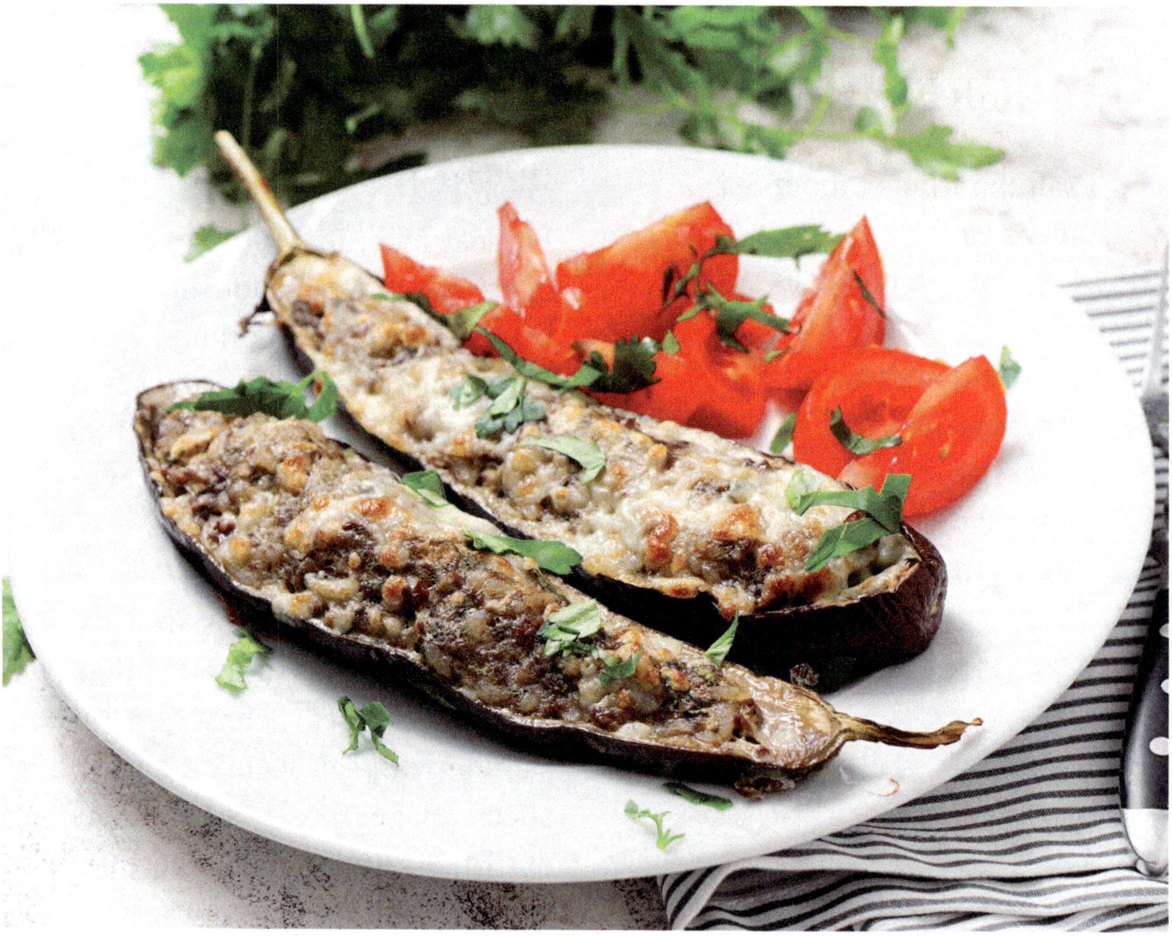

NUTRITIONAL INFORMATION

Calories 400, Fat 20g, Carbs 25g, Protein 30g

INGREDIENTS

- 1 large eggplant
- 1 pound ground chicken
- 1 cup chopped mushrooms
- 1/2 onion, chopped
- 1 clove garlic, minced
- 1 tablespoon olive oil
- 1/2 teaspoon dried oregano
- 1/4 teaspoon salt
- 1/4 teaspoon black pepper
- 1/4 cup shredded vegan mozzarella cheese (optional)

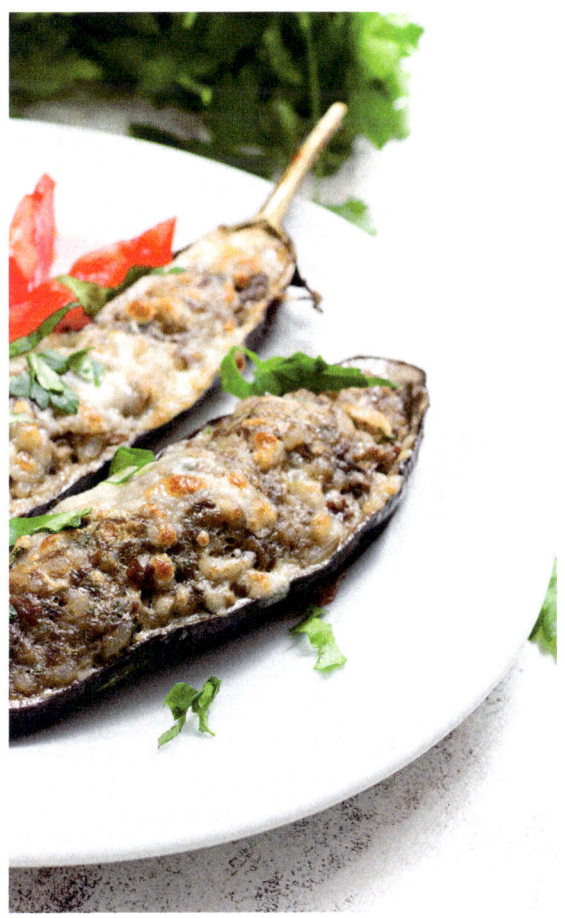

DESCRIPTION

STEP 1
Preheat oven to 375 degrees F (190 degrees C). Cut the eggplant in half lengthwise and scoop out the flesh, leaving a 1/2-inch shell. Chop the eggplant flesh and set aside.

STEP 2
In a large skillet, heat the olive oil over medium heat. Add the onion and cook until softened, about 5 minutes. Add the garlic and cook for 30 seconds more, until fragrant.

STEP 3
Add the ground chicken and cook, breaking it up with a spoon, until browned. Drain off any excess grease. Stir in the chopped mushrooms, oregano, salt, and pepper. Cook for 5 minutes more, or until the mushrooms are tender.

STEP 4
Stir in the reserved chopped eggplant flesh. Divide the chicken mixture among the eggplant halves. Sprinkle with mozzarella cheese. Bake for 20-25 minutes, or until the eggplants are tender.

CARROT & ALMOND SALAD

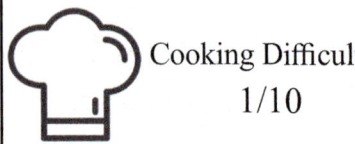 Cooking Difficulty: 1/10	 Cooking Time: 3 minutes	 Servings: 2

INGREDIENTS

- 2 medium carrots, grated
- 2 tablespoons almonds, chopped
- 1 tablespoon olive oil
- 1 teaspoon lemon juice
- salt and pepper, to taste

DESCRIPTION

STEP 1
Toss grated carrots and chopped almonds in a bowl. Drizzle with olive oil and lemon juice, season with salt and pepper, and mix. Serve and enjoy!

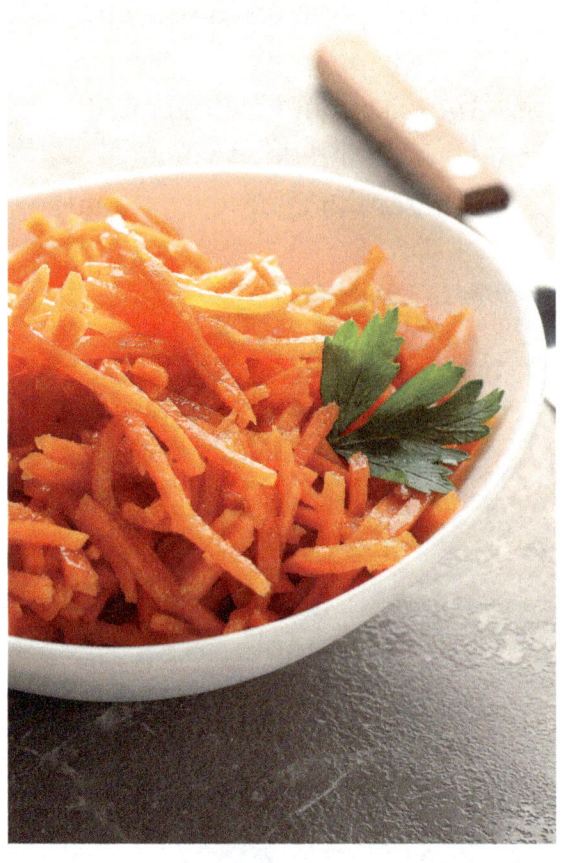

NUTRITIONAL INFORMATION

70 Calories, 0g Fat, 2g Carbs, 1g Protein

RADISH & AVOCADO SALAD

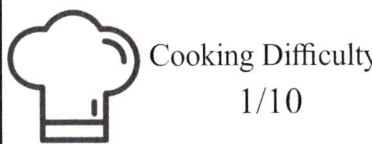 Cooking Difficulty: 1/10

 Cooking Time: 3 minutes

 Servings: 2

INGREDIENTS

- 1/2 bunch radishes, thinly sliced
- 1 avocado, diced
- 1/2 cup mixed microgreens
- 2 cups mixed salad greens
- 1 tablespoon olive oil
- salt and pepper, to taste

DESCRIPTION

STEP 1
Combine radishes, microgreens, avocado, and salad greens in a bowl. Drizzle with olive oil, season with salt and pepper, and toss gently. Serve and enjoy!

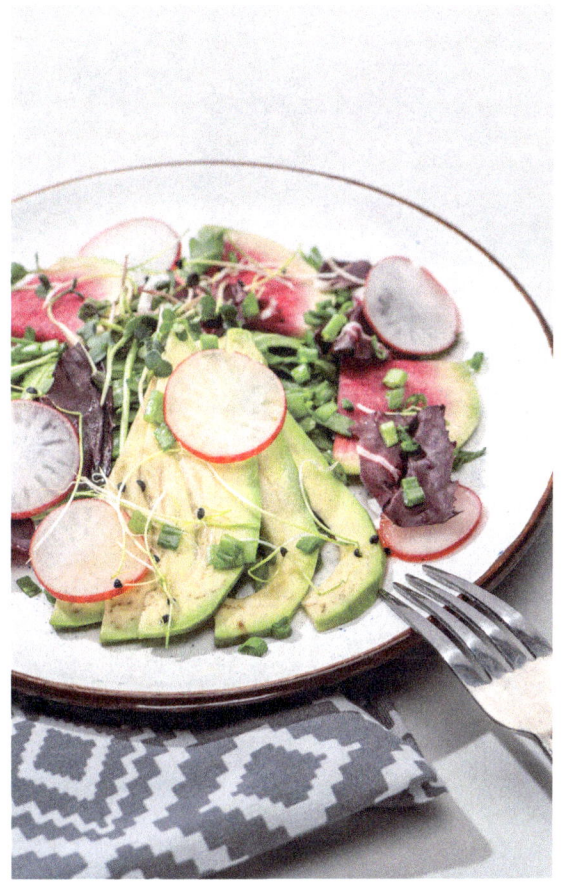

NUTRITIONAL INFORMATION
95 Calories, 2g Fat, 4g Carbs, 2g Protein

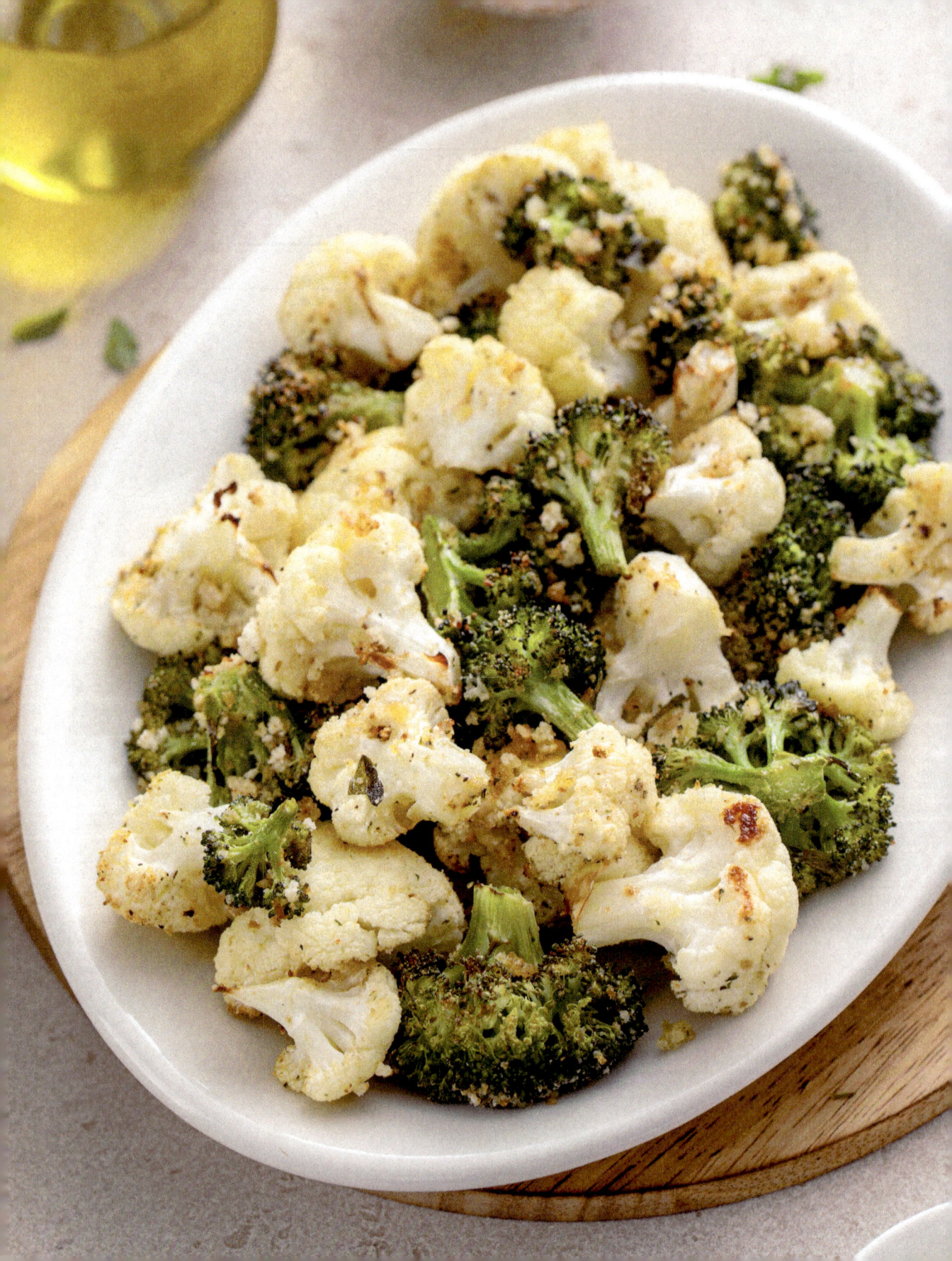

VEGGIE ROAST

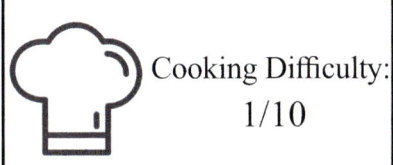 Cooking Difficulty: 1/10
 Cooking Time: 30 minutes
 Servings: 2

INGREDIENTS

- 1 cup broccoli florets
- 1 cup cauliflower florets
- 2 tablespoons olive oil
- 1/2 teaspoon salt
- 1/4 teaspoon black pepper
- 1/4 teaspoon paprika

DESCRIPTION

STEP 1
Preheat oven to 400 degrees F (200 degrees C). In a large bowl, toss broccoli, cauliflower, olive oil, salt, pepper, and paprika.

STEP 2
Spread vegetables in a single layer on a baking sheet lined with parchment paper.

STEP 3
Roast for 20-25 minutes, or until vegetables are tender and slightly crispy.

NUTRITIONAL INFORMATION

Calories: 150, Fat: 10g, Carbs: 10g, Protein: 5g

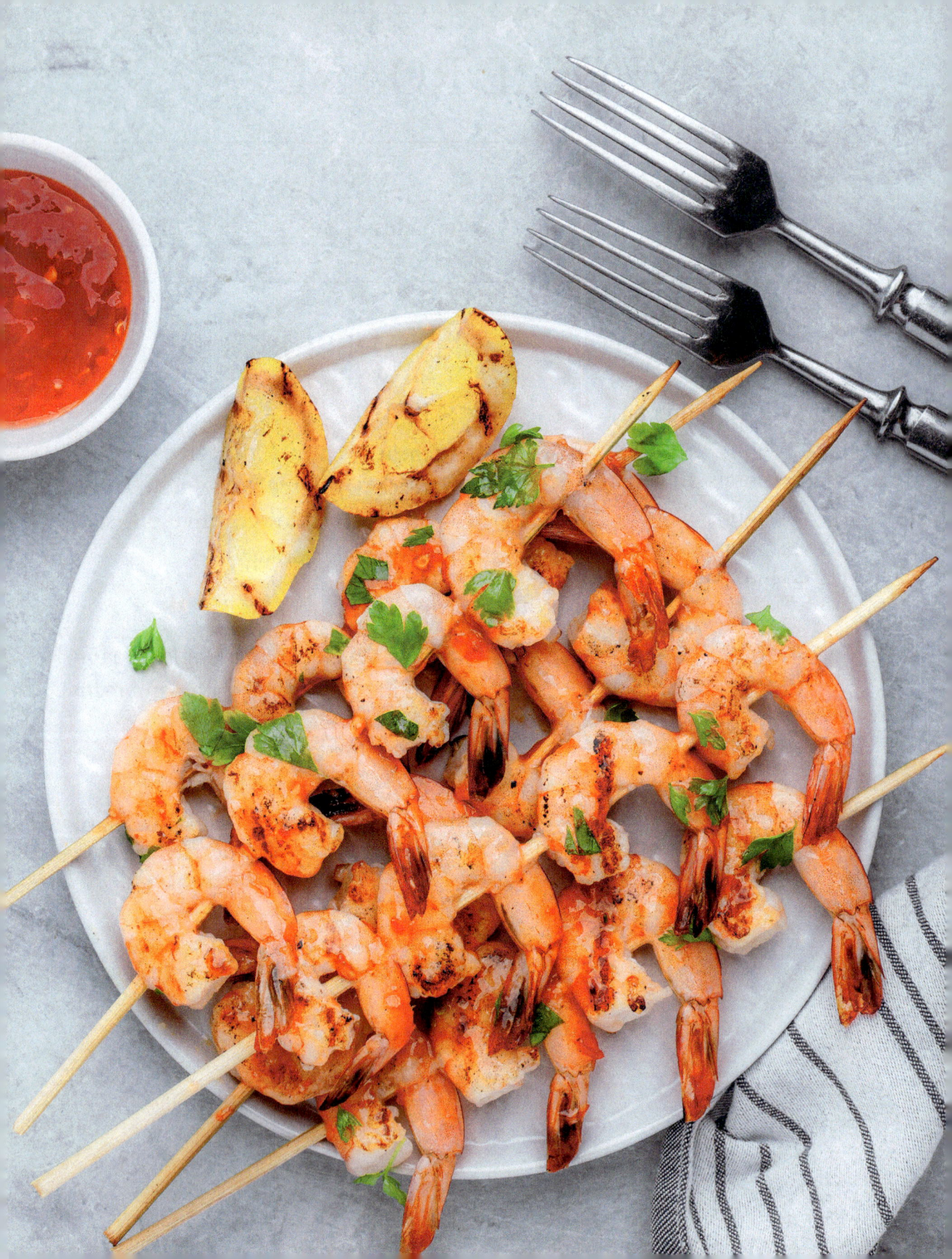

GRILLED SHRIMP SKEWERS

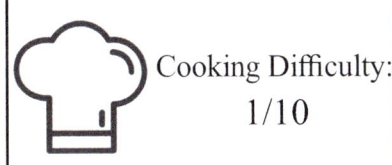 Cooking Difficulty: 1/10

 Cooking Time: 38 minutes

 Servings: 2

INGREDIENTS

- 1 pound large shrimp, tails on and unpeeled
- ¼ cup olive oil
- 2 tablespoons lime juice
- 1 tablespoon minced garlic
- 1 teaspoon dried oregano
- ½ teaspoon salt
- ¼ teaspoon black pepper
- ¼ cup chopped fresh parsley (optional)

DESCRIPTION

STEP 1
In a medium bowl, whisk together olive oil, lime juice, garlic, oregano, salt, and pepper. Add shrimp and toss to coat. Cover and refrigerate for 30 minutes, or up to 2 hours.

STEP 2
Preheat grill pan or grill to medium heat. Thread shrimp onto skewers, leaving tails on. Grill for 2-3 minutes per side, or until shrimp are pink and opaque.

STEP 3
Serve shrimp skewers immediately with lemon wedges and fresh herbs.

NUTRITIONAL INFORMATION

Calories: 350, Fat: 15g, Carbs: 5g, Protein: 35g

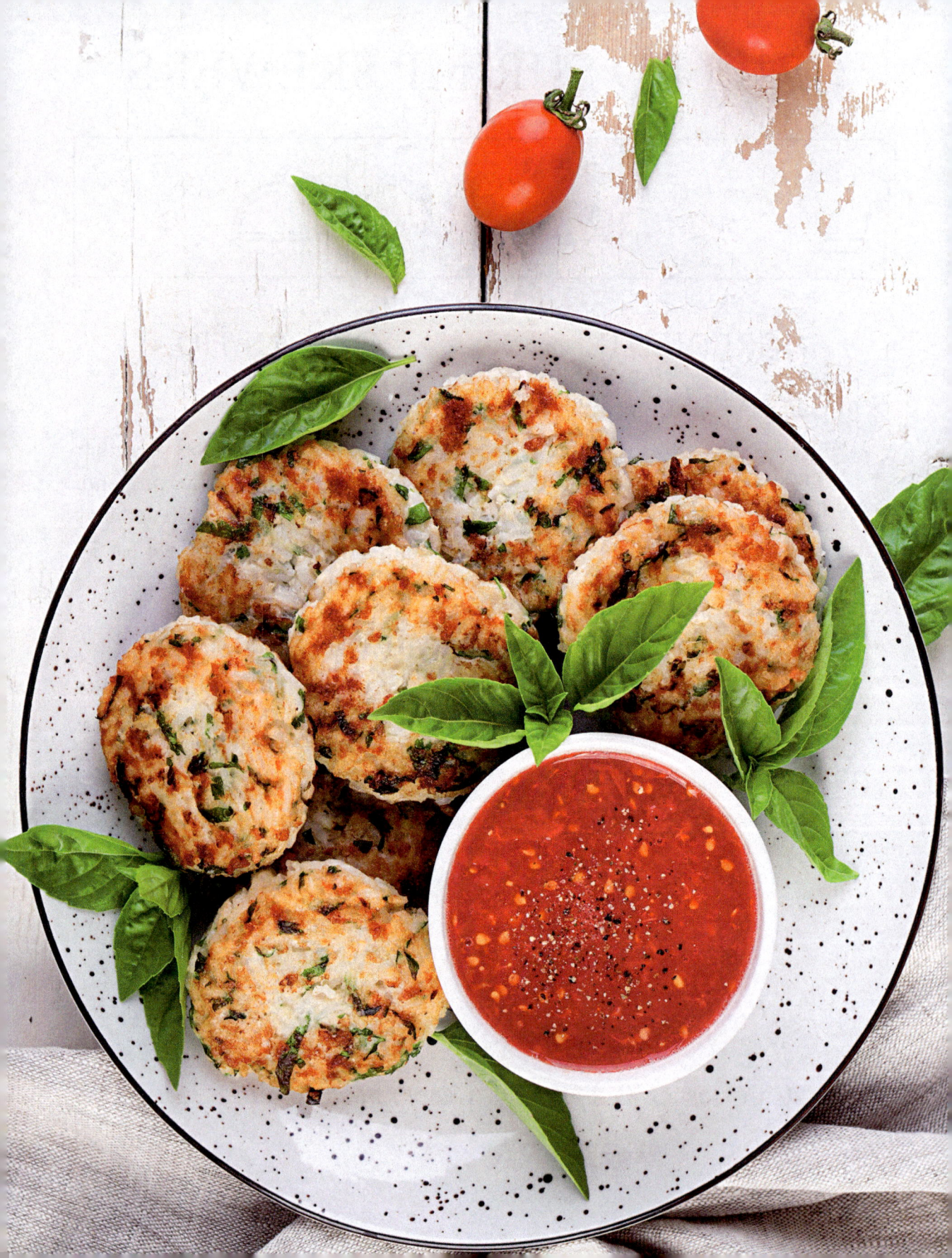

CHICKEN PATTIES

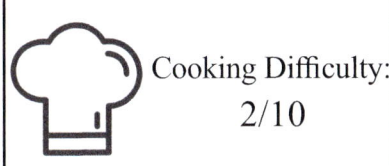 Cooking Difficulty: 2/10

 Cooking Time: 28 minutes

 Servings: 2

INGREDIENTS

- 10.5 oz (300 g) ground chicken
- 3.5 oz (100 g) spinach, chopped
- ¼ cup (1/2 onion) finely chopped
- 1 egg
- 2 tablespoons rolled oats
- 1 tablespoon olive oil
- salt and pepper to taste

DESCRIPTION

STEP 1
Preheat oven to 350°F (180°C).

STEP 2
In a bowl, combine chicken, spinach, onion, egg, oats, olive oil, salt, and pepper. Shape mixture into 2 meatballs. Place meatballs on a baking sheet lined with parchment paper.

STEP 3
Bake for 20-25 minutes, or until meatballs are cooked through.

NUTRITIONAL INFORMATION

350 Calories, 15g Fat, 10g Carbs, 30g Protein

CHICKEN MEATBALL SOUP

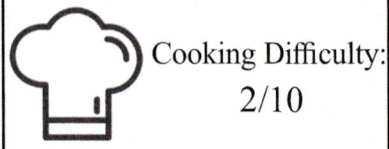 Cooking Difficulty: 2/10	 Cooking Time: 40 minutes	 Servings: 3

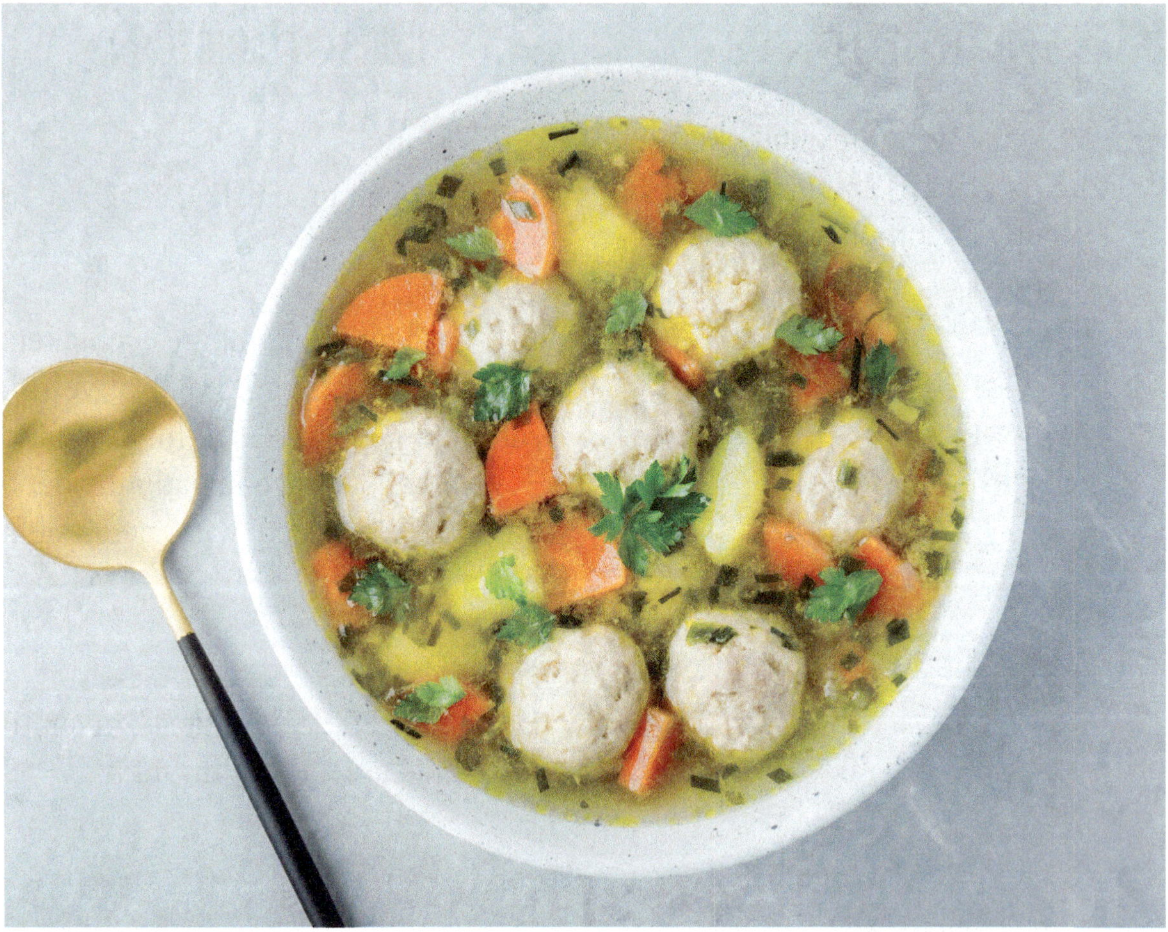

NUTRITIONAL INFORMATION

Calories 350, Fat 15g, Carbs 30g, Protein 25g

INGREDIENTS

for the meatballs:
- 1 pound ground chicken
- 1 onion, finely chopped
- 1 egg
- 2 tablespoons breadcrumbs
- 1 tablespoon milk
- salt and pepper to taste

for the soup:
- 8 cups vegetable broth
- 3 potatoes, diced
- 2 carrots, diced
- 1 bay leaf
- 3-4 black peppercorns
- salt and pepper to taste
- fresh herbs for garnish (optional)

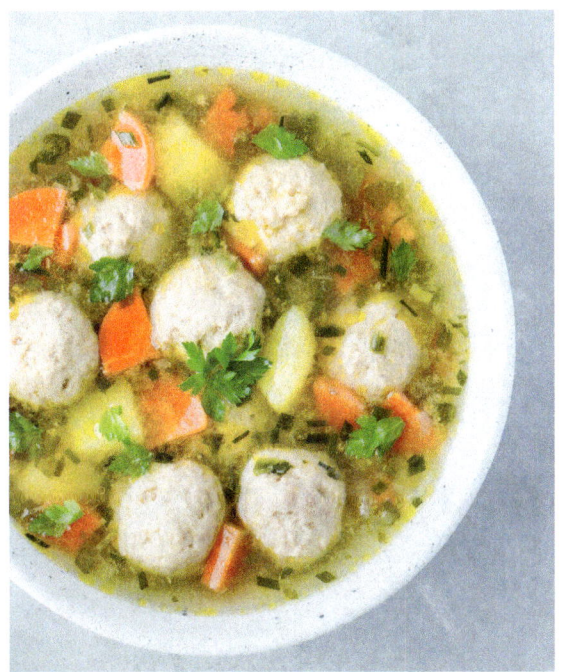

DESCRIPTION

STEP 1
In a bowl, combine the ground chicken, onion, egg, breadcrumbs, milk, salt, and pepper. Mix well until the mixture is evenly distributed. Shape the mixture into small meatballs.

STEP 2
In a large pot, bring the vegetable broth to a boil. Add the potatoes, carrots, bay leaf, and black peppercorns. Cook for 10-15 minutes, or until the vegetables are tender.

STEP 3
Gently drop the meatballs into the simmering soup and cook for an additional 10-15 minutes, or until the meatballs are cooked through and float to the top. Season with salt and pepper to taste.

STEP 4
Ladle the soup into bowls and garnish with fresh herbs, if desired.

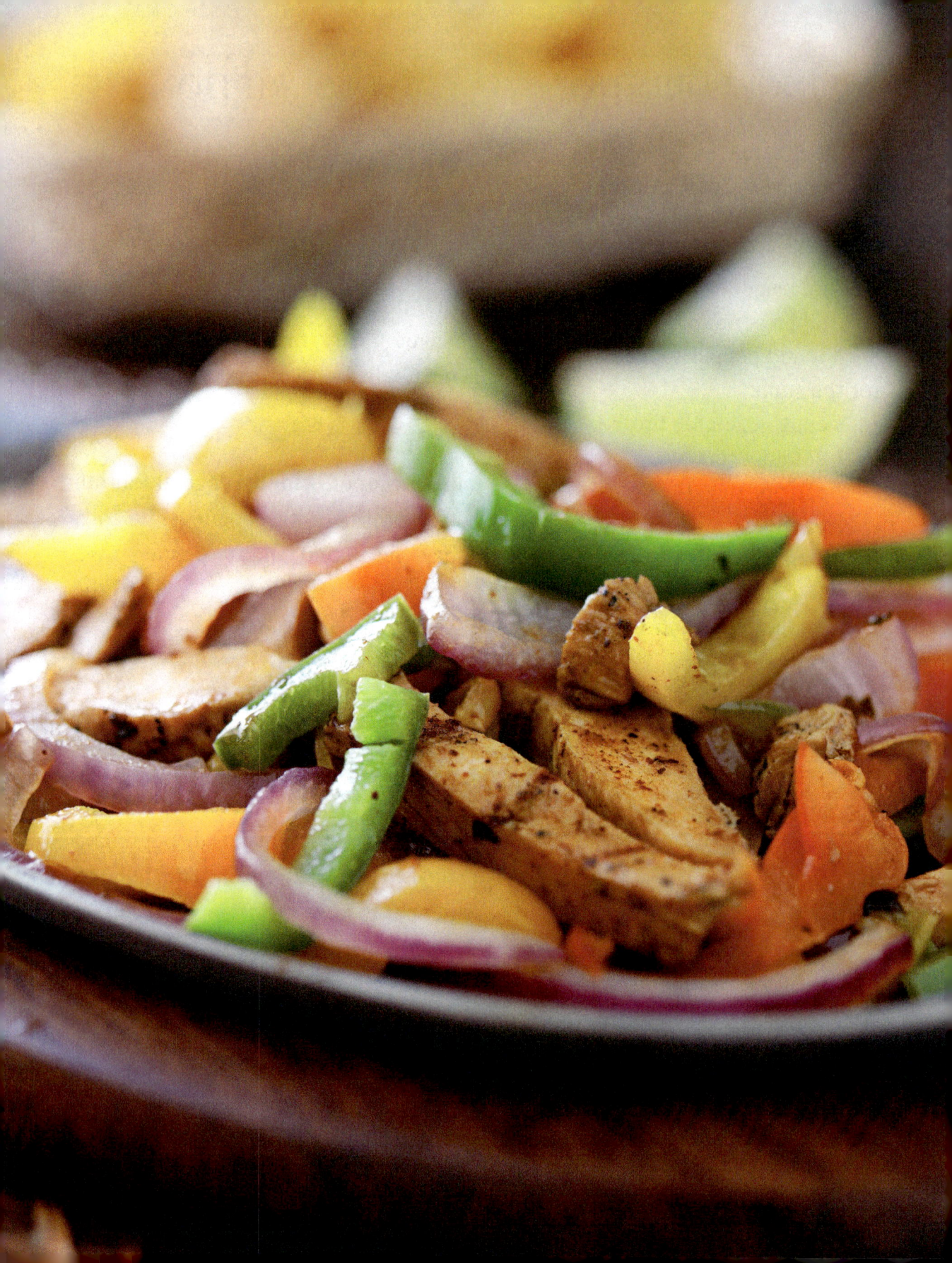

CHICKEN WITH VEGETABLES

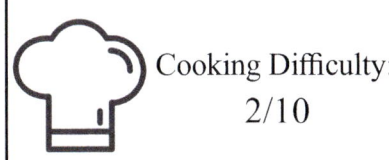 Cooking Difficulty: 2/10

 Cooking Time: 18 minutes

 Servings: 2

INGREDIENTS

- 1 oz anchovies in oil
- 1 oz kalamata olives
- 2.5 oz cherry tomatoes
- 1/4 red onion, thinly sliced
- 2.5 oz spinach
- 1 hard-boiled egg, sliced
- 1 tablespoon olive oil
- 1 tablespoon lemon juice
- salt and pepper to taste

DESCRIPTION

STEP 1
Heat olive oil in a large skillet over medium heat.

STEP 2
Add chicken and cook until golden brown and cooked through, about 5-7 minutes per side. Add zucchini, bell pepper, and red onion to the pan. Cook for an additional 5-7 minutes, or until vegetables are tender-crisp. Season with salt and pepper to taste.

STEP 3
Serve immediately.

NUTRITIONAL INFORMATION

350 Calories, 15g Fat, 10g Carbs, 30g Protein

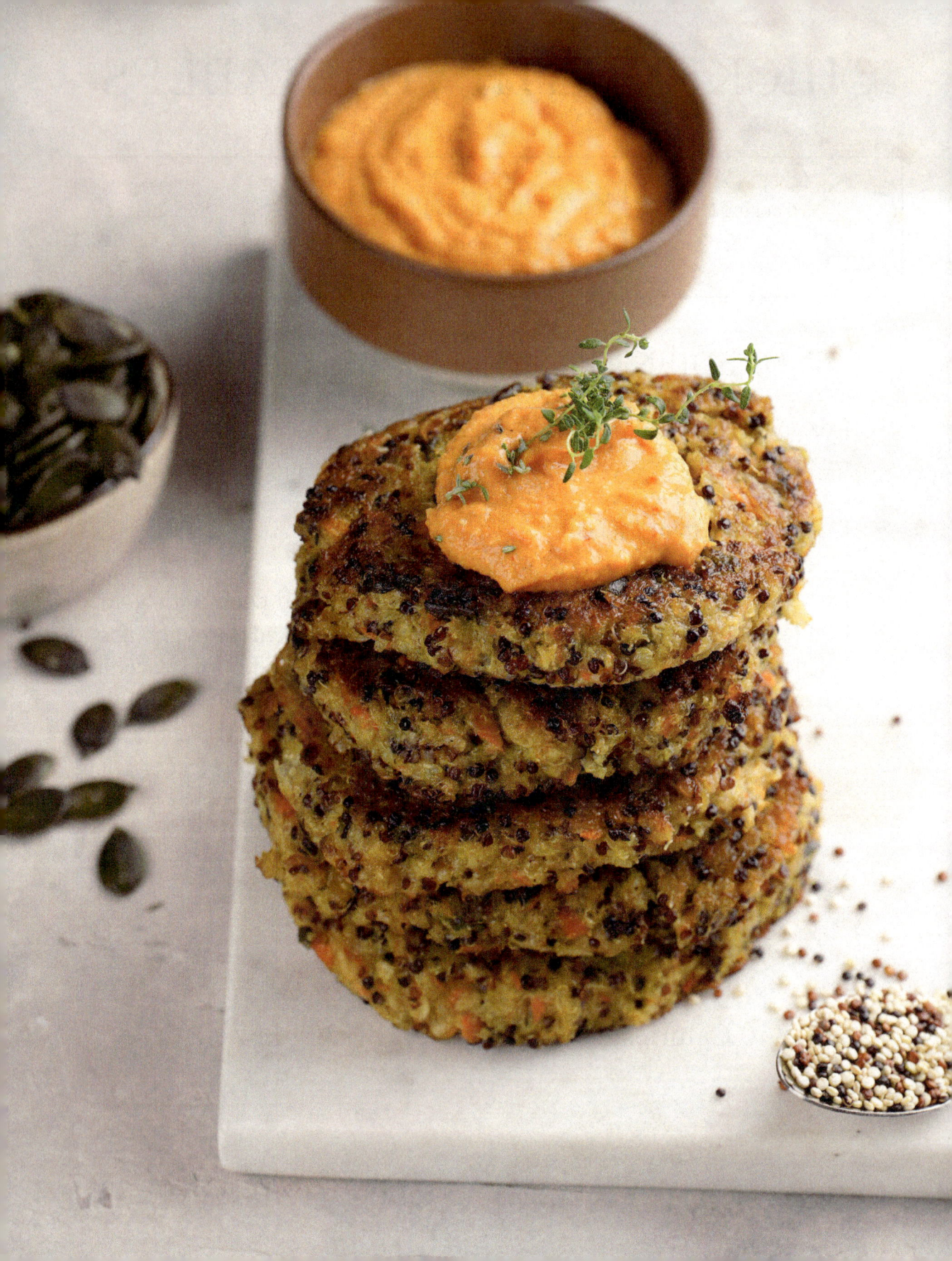

QUINOA VEGGIE PATTIES

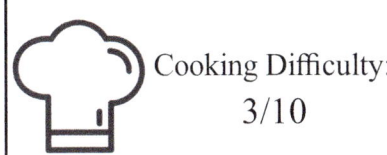 Cooking Difficulty: 3/10

 Cooking Time: 18 minutes

 Servings: 2

INGREDIENTS

- 1/2 cup quinoa, rinsed
- 1 cup water
- 1 medium carrot, grated
- 1/2 red onion, finely chopped
- 1 clove garlic, minced
- 1/2 cup cooked chickpeas, mashed
- 2 tablespoons chopped fresh parsley
- salt and pepper to taste
- 1 egg
- 2 tablespoons breadcrumbs or flour
- 2 tablespoons olive oil

DESCRIPTION

STEP 1
Cook quinoa in water until all water is absorbed. In a large bowl, combine cooked quinoa, mashed chickpeas, grated carrot, chopped onion, minced garlic, parsley, salt, pepper, and egg. Add breadcrumbs or flour to help the mixture bind together.

STEP 2
Form the mixture into patties. Heat olive oil in a skillet over medium heat. Cook the patties in the skillet until golden brown on both sides.

STEP 3
Serve hot with your favorite sauce. Enjoy!

NUTRITIONAL INFORMATION

Calories: 280, Fat: 14g, Carbs: 28g, Protein: 12g

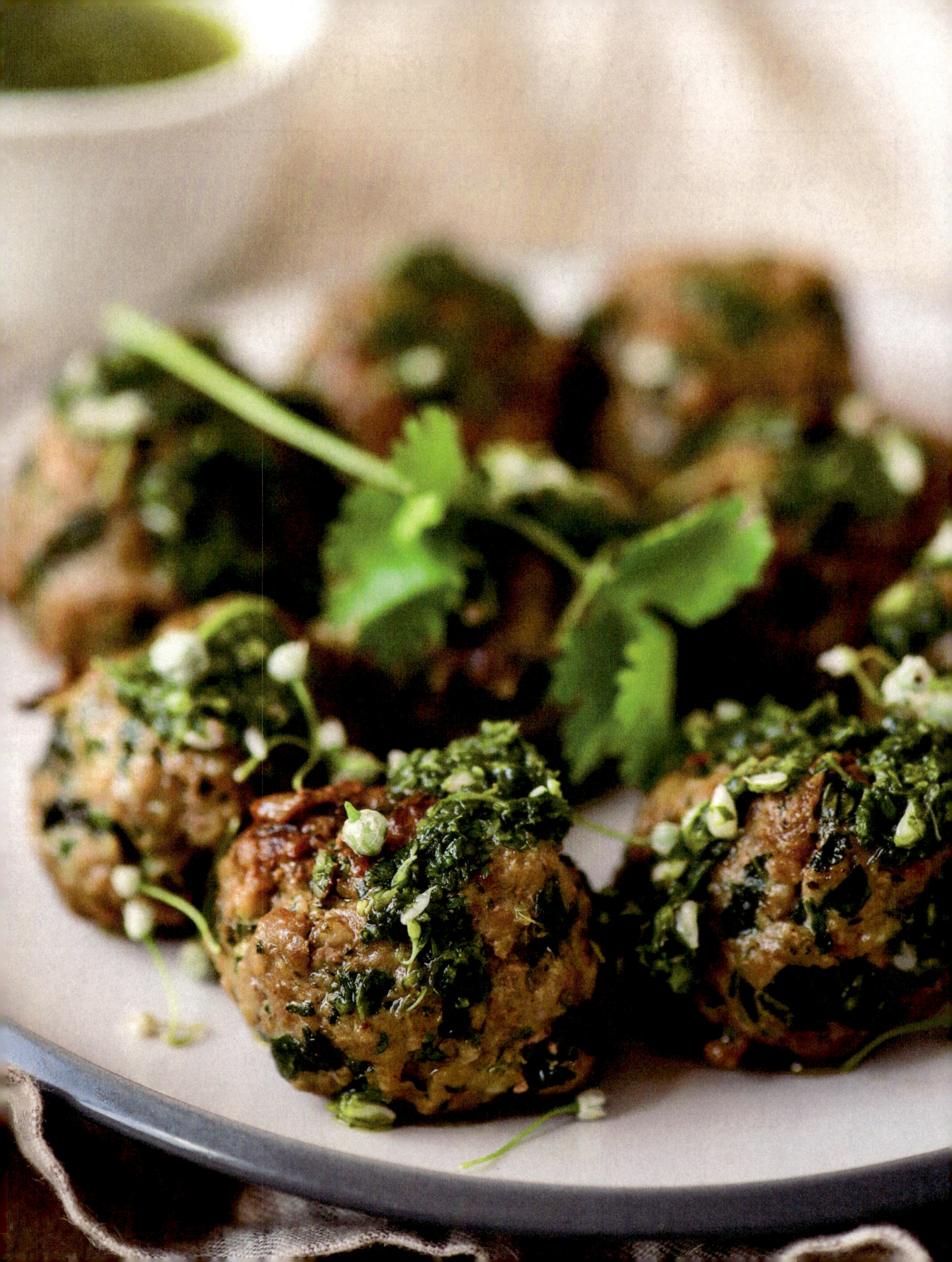

TURKEY MEATBALLS WITH MINT

 Cooking Difficulty: 2/10

 Cooking Time: 27 minutes

 Servings: 4

INGREDIENTS

- 1 pound ground turkey
- 1/2 onion, finely chopped
- 1 clove garlic, minced
- 1/4 cup fresh mint, chopped
- 1/4 cup fresh spinach leaves, chopped
- 1 egg
- 1/4 cup bread crumbs
- 1 tablespoon olive oil
- 1/2 teaspoon salt
- 1/4 teaspoon black pepper
- 1/4 teaspoon nutmeg

DESCRIPTION

STEP 1
Preheat oven to 350 degrees F (175 degrees C). In a large bowl, combine turkey, onion, garlic, mint, spinach, egg, bread crumbs, olive oil, salt, pepper, and nutmeg.

STEP 2
Shape the mixture into 1-inch meatballs. Place meatballs on a baking sheet lined with parchment paper. Bake for 20-25 minutes, or until meatballs are browned and cooked through.

STEP 3
Serve with your favorite sauce, such as tomato sauce, yogurt sauce, or pesto.

NUTRITIONAL INFORMATION

Calories: 350, Fat: 15g, Carbs: 10g, Protein: 35g

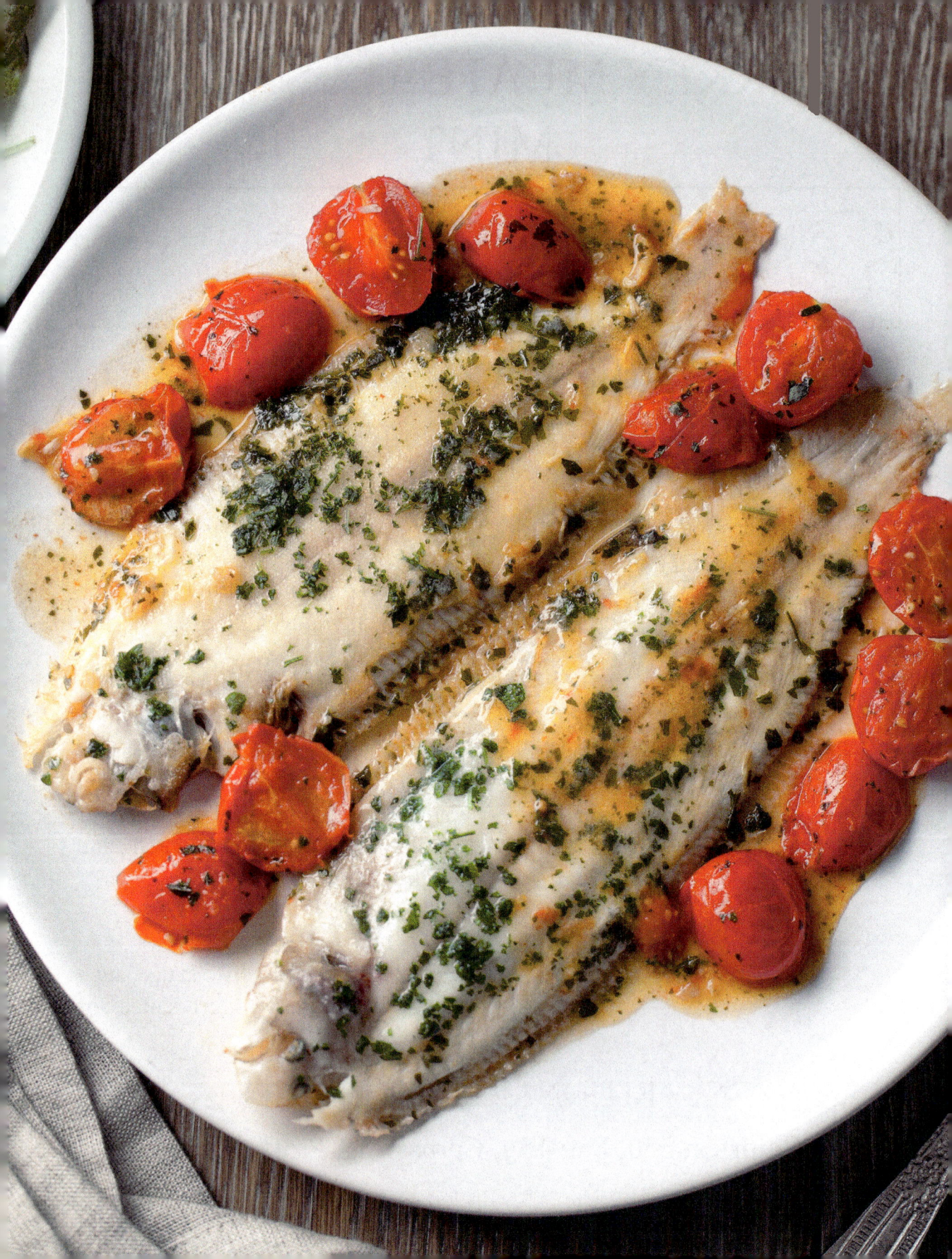

STEAMED WHITE FISH WITH TOMATOES

 Cooking Difficulty: 3/10

 Cooking Time: 18 minutes

 Servings: 2

INGREDIENTS

- 5.3 oz (150 g) white fish fillets (hake, cod, or pollock; 2 pieces)
- 1 tomato, diced
- ¼ cup (1/2 onion) diced
- 1 tablespoon olive oil
- 1 teaspoon lemon juice
- salt and pepper to taste

DESCRIPTION

STEP 1
Bring water to a boil in a saucepan. Place a steamer basket over the boiling water.

STEP 2
Arrange fish fillets on the steamer basket. Top with tomatoes and onion. Steam for 10-15 minutes, or until fish is opaque and vegetables are tender.

STEP 3
Drizzle with olive oil, lemon juice, season with salt and pepper to taste.

NUTRITIONAL INFORMATION

Calories: 210, Fat: 10g, Carbs: 8g, Protein: 12g

CHICKPEA SALAD

 Cooking Difficulty: 1/10    Cooking Time: 3 minutes   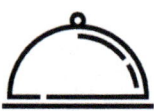 Servings: 2

INGREDIENTS

- 1 cups fresh spinach
- 1 cup canned chickpeas, drained and rinsed
- 1 ripe avocado, diced
- 1/2 cucumber, diced
- 1/4 cup cherry tomatoes, halved
- 1 tablespoon fresh lemon juice
- 1 tablespoon olive oil
- salt and pepper, to taste

DESCRIPTION

STEP 1
In a bowl, mix chickpeas, avocado, spinach, cucumber, and tomatoes. Add lemon juice, olive oil, salt, and pepper. Toss gently and enjoy!

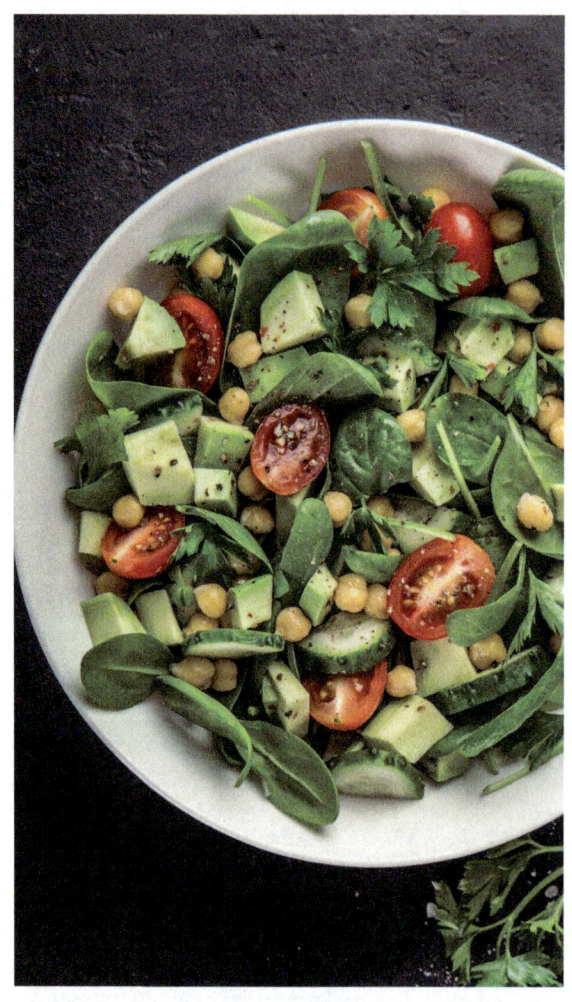

NUTRITIONAL INFORMATION
116 Calories, 2g Fat, 7g Carbs, 5g Protein

APPLE SPINACH SALAD

 Cooking Difficulty: 1/10

 Cooking Time: 4 minutes

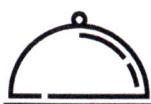 Servings: 2

INGREDIENTS

- 2 cups fresh spinach
- 1 apple, thinly sliced
- 2 tablespoons walnuts, chopped
- 1 tablespoon olive oil
- 1 teaspoon apple cider vinegar
- salt and pepper, to taste

DESCRIPTION

STEP 1

In a bowl, combine spinach, apple slices, and walnuts. Drizzle with olive oil and apple cider vinegar, season with salt and pepper, toss gently, and enjoy!

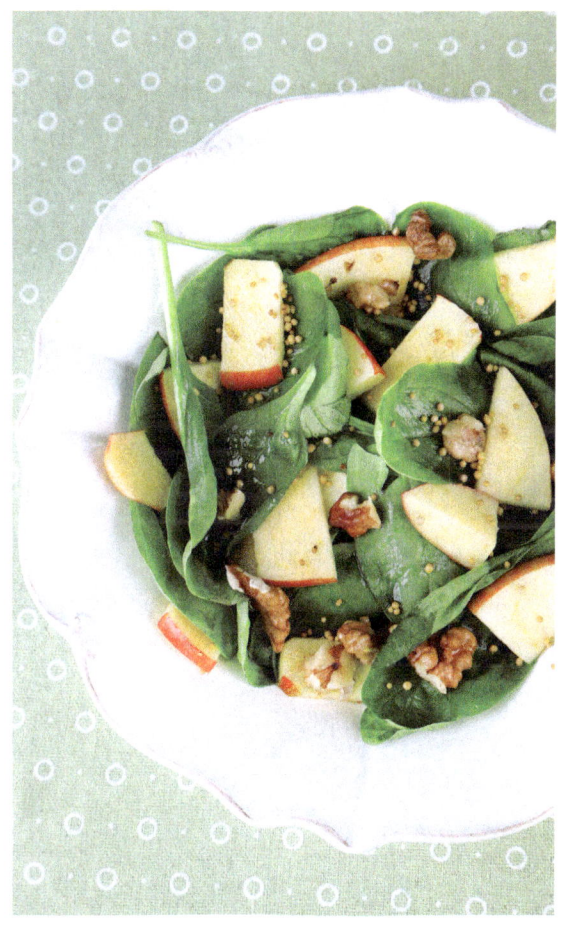

NUTRITIONAL INFORMATION

89 Calories, 3g Fat, 4g Carbs, 2g Protein

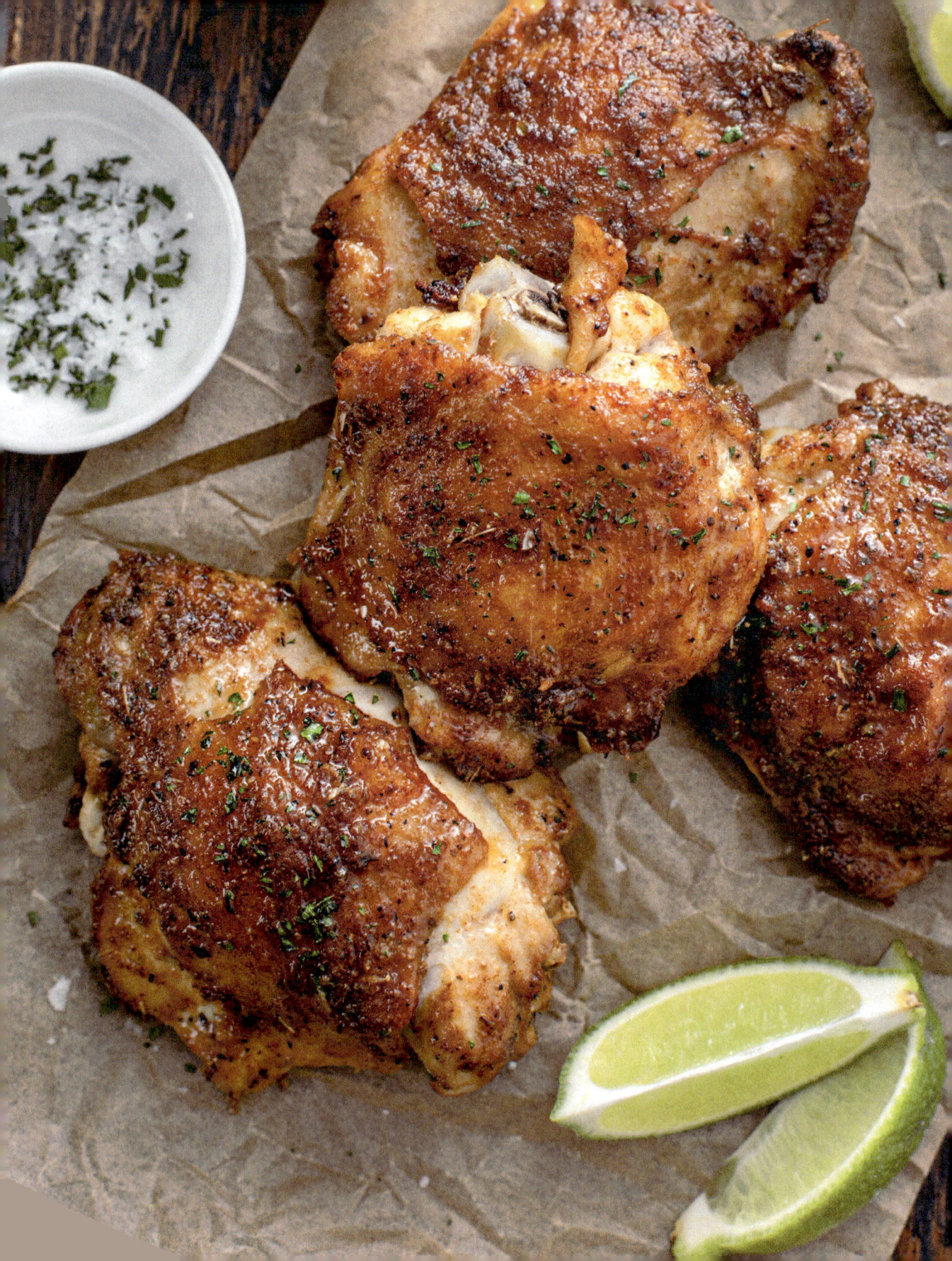

AROMATIC CHICKEN THIGHS WITH HERBS

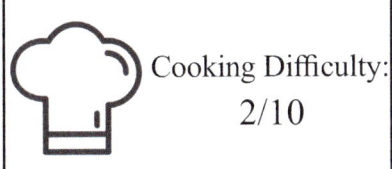 Cooking Difficulty: 2/10

 Cooking Time: 45 minutes

 Servings: 4

INGREDIENTS

- 4 chicken thighs (about 1 pound)
- 2 tablespoons olive oil
- 1 teaspoon salt
- 1/2 teaspoon black pepper
- 1/2 teaspoon paprika
- 1/4 teaspoon garlic powder
- 1/4 teaspoon onion powder
- 1/4 teaspoon smoked paprika
- 1/4 teaspoon ground cumin
- 1/8 teaspoon cayenne pepper (optional)
- 1/4 cup fresh parsley, chopped

DESCRIPTION

STEP 1
Preheat oven to 400 degrees F (200 degrees C). In a small bowl, combine olive oil, salt, pepper, paprika, garlic powder, onion powder, smoked paprika, cumin, and cayenne pepper (optional). Rub the spice mixture all over the chicken thighs.

STEP 2
Place the chicken thighs on a baking sheet lined with parchment paper. Roast for 35-45 minutes, or until the chicken is cooked through and the juices run clear. Sprinkle with parsley and serve.

NUTRITIONAL INFORMATION

Calories: 400, Fat: 25g, Carbs: 5g, Protein: 30g

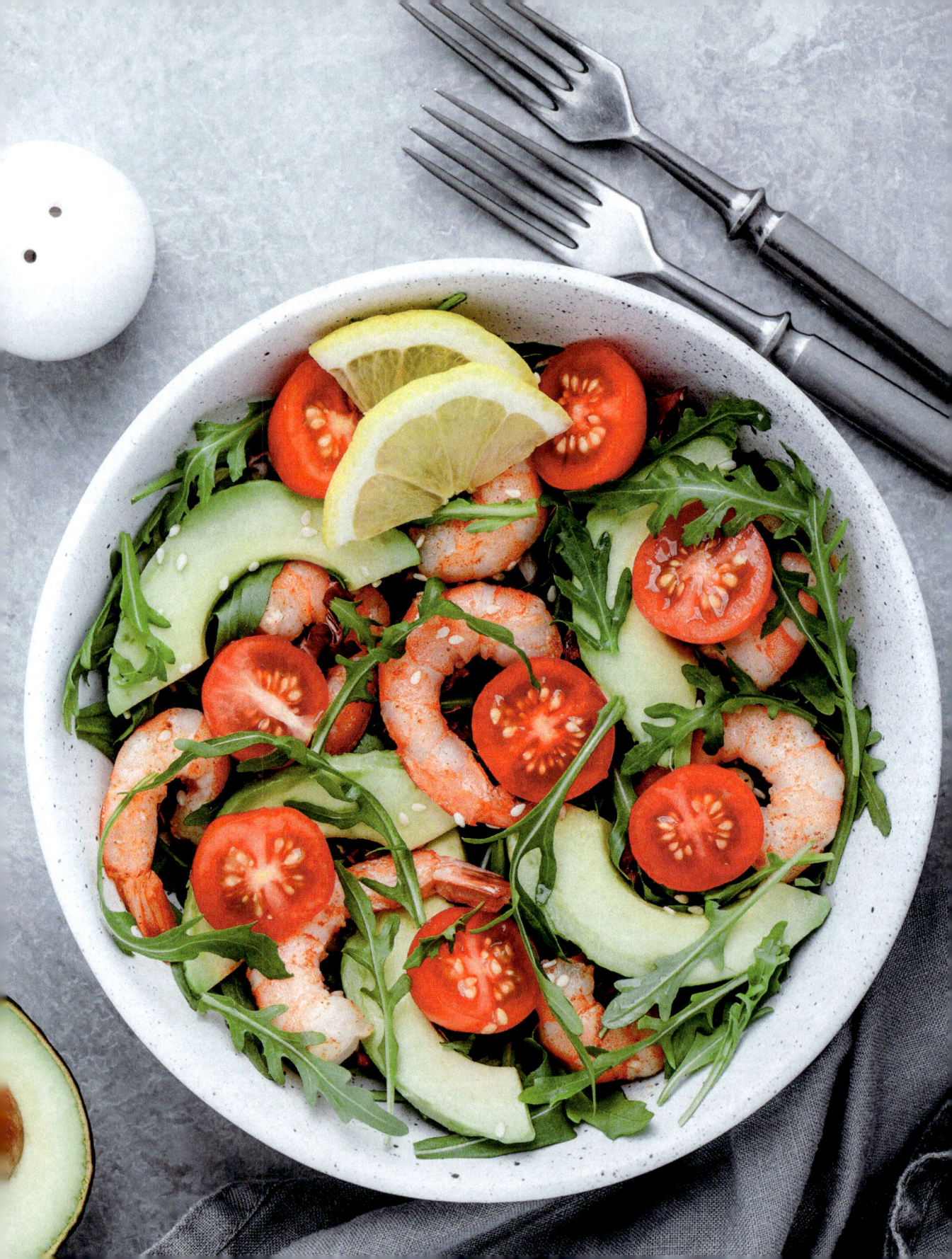

AVOCADO, CHERRY TOMATO, SHRIMP, AND ARUGULA SALAD

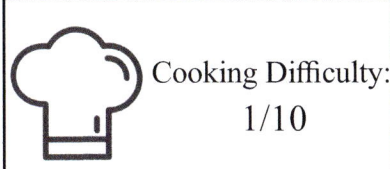 Cooking Difficulty: 1/10

 Cooking Time: 5 minutes

 Servings: 2

INGREDIENTS

for the salad:
- 4 cups baby arugula
- 1 ripe avocado, halved, pitted, and sliced
- 1 cup cherry tomatoes, halved
- 12 cooked and peeled shrimp

for the vinaigrette:
- 2 tablespoons olive oil
- 1 tablespoon lemon juice
- 1 teaspoon dijon mustard
- 1/2 teaspoon dried oregano
- salt and pepper to taste

DESCRIPTION

STEP 1
In a small bowl, whisk together the olive oil, lemon juice, Dijon mustard, oregano, salt, and pepper. Set aside.

STEP 2
In a large bowl, combine the arugula, avocado, cherry tomatoes, and shrimp.

STEP 3
Drizzle the vinaigrette over the salad and toss gently to coat.

STEP 4
Serve immediately and enjoy!

NUTRITIONAL INFORMATION

Calories: 200, Fat: 15g, Carbs: 17g, Protein: 24g

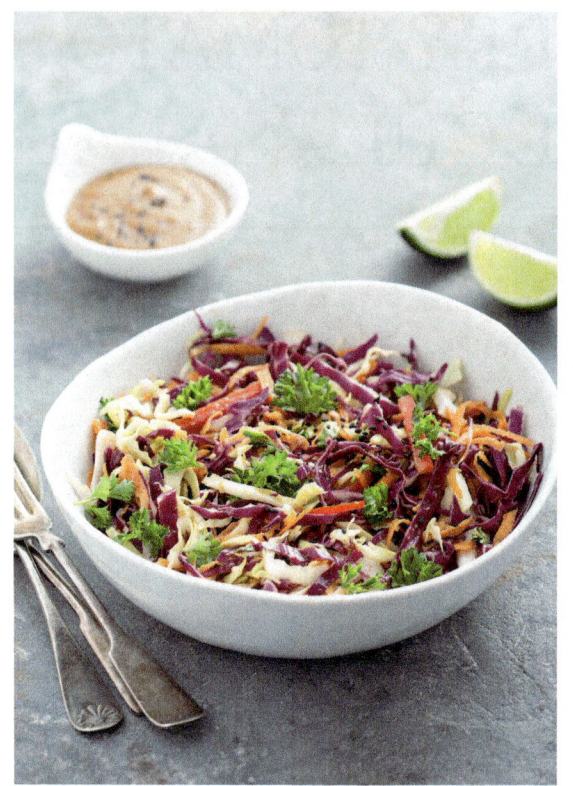
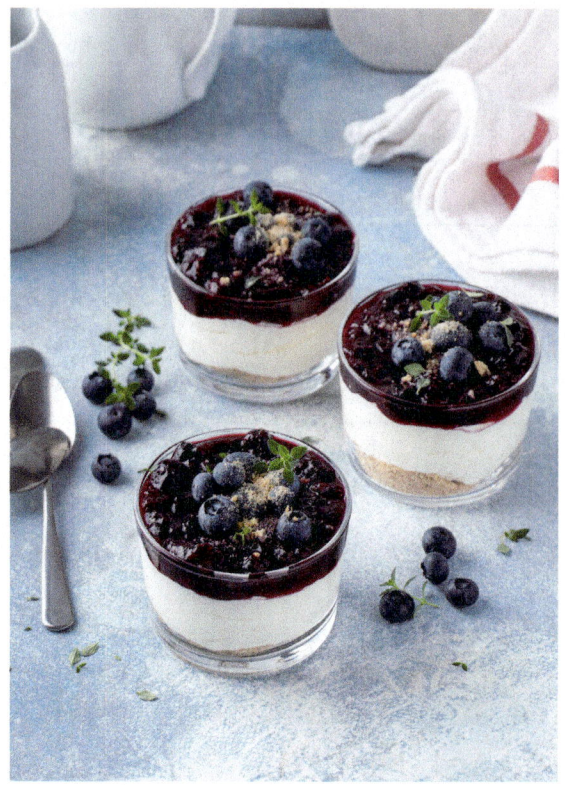
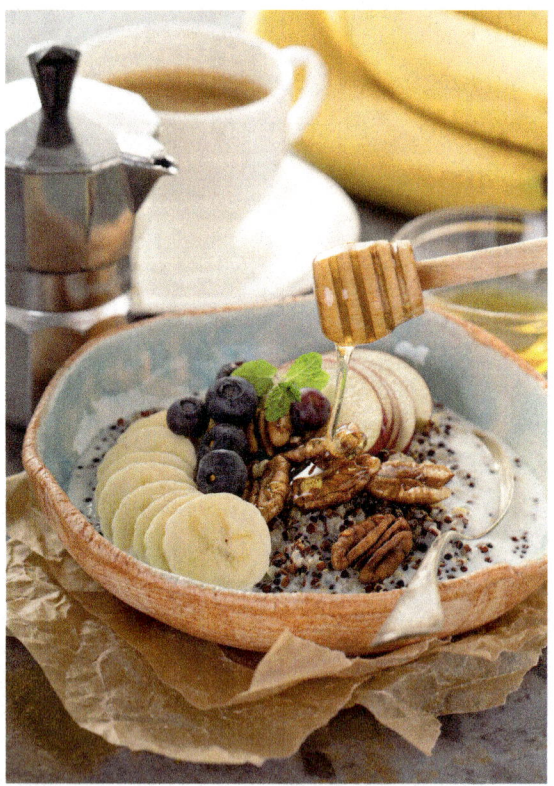
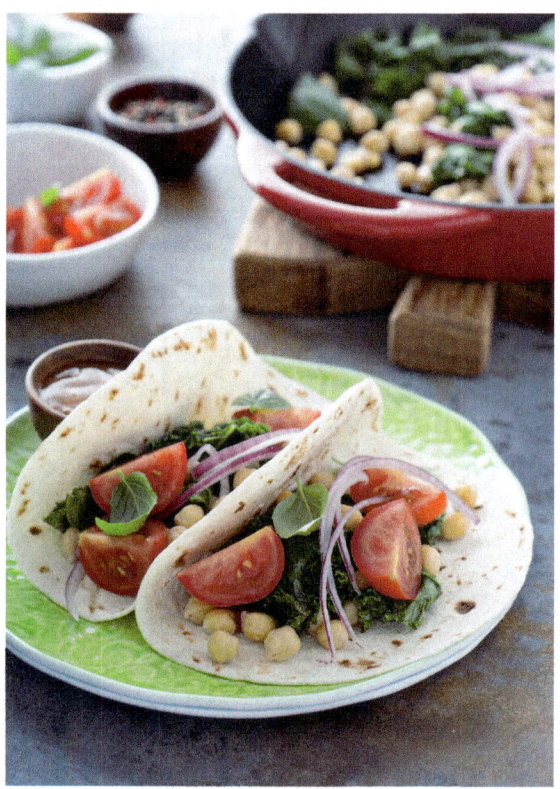

SNACKS & DESSERTS

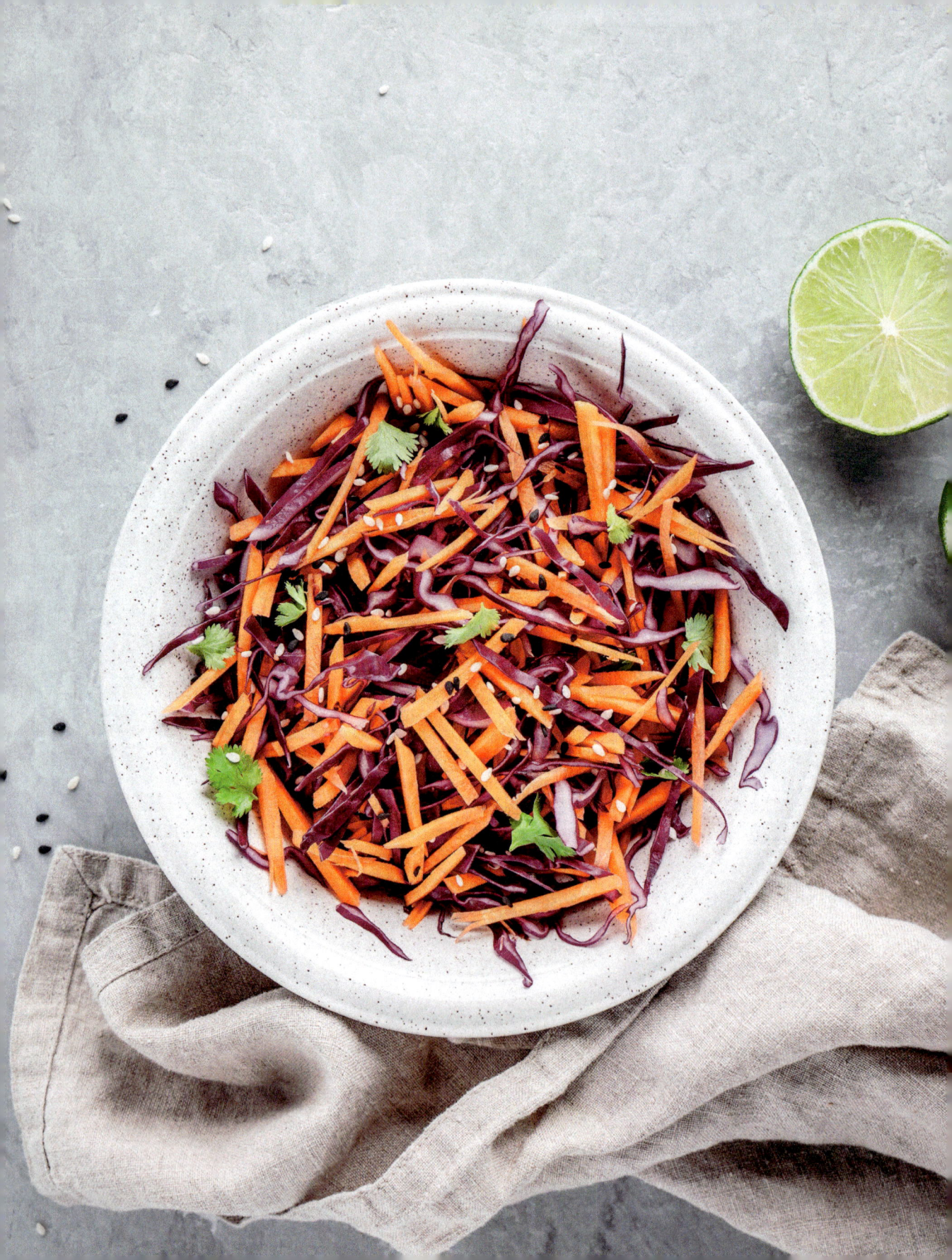

CARROT AND RED CABBAGE SALAD

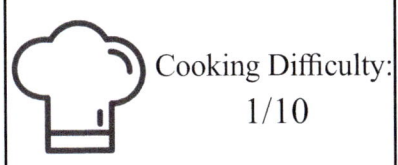 Cooking Difficulty: 1/10

 Cooking Time: 5 minutes

 Servings: 2

INGREDIENTS

- 2 cups shredded carrots
- 2 cups shredded red cabbage
- 1/4 cup chopped fresh parsley
- 2 tablespoons olive oil
- 1 tablespoon lemon juice
- salt and pepper to taste

DESCRIPTION

STEP 1
In a large bowl, combine the shredded carrots, red cabbage, and parsley.

STEP 2
In a small bowl, whisk together the olive oil, lemon juice, salt, and pepper.

STEP 3
Pour the dressing over the salad and toss to coat. Serve immediately.

NUTRITIONAL INFORMATION

Calories: 200, Fat: 10g, Carbs: 20g, Protein: 2g

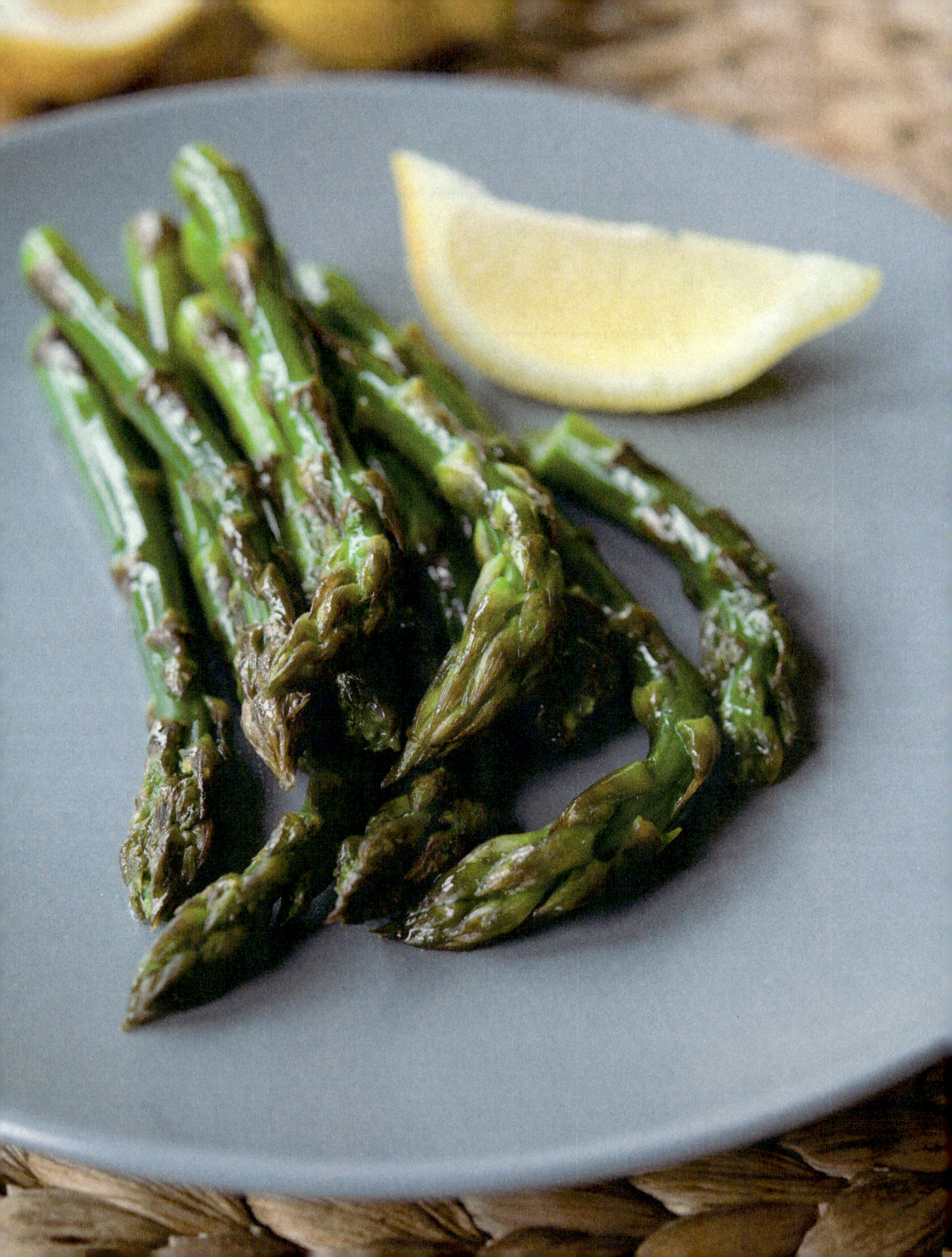

ASPARAGUS SPEARS

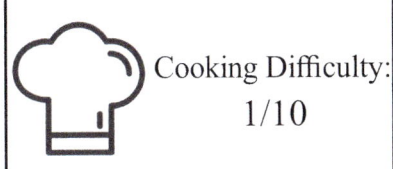 Cooking Difficulty: 1/10

 Cooking Time: 12 minutes

 Servings: 2

INGREDIENTS

- 8.8 oz (250 g) fresh asparagus
- 1 tablespoon olive oil
- salt and pepper to taste

DESCRIPTION

STEP 1
Preheat oven to 400°F (200°C).

STEP 2
Line a baking sheet with parchment paper. 3. Wash asparagus and trim off the tough ends. Arrange asparagus on the prepared baking sheet. Drizzle asparagus with olive oil, season with salt and pepper to taste.

STEP 3
Roast for 10 minutes, or until asparagus is tender.

NUTRITIONAL INFORMATION

70 Calories, 3g Fat, 9g Carbs, 4g Protein

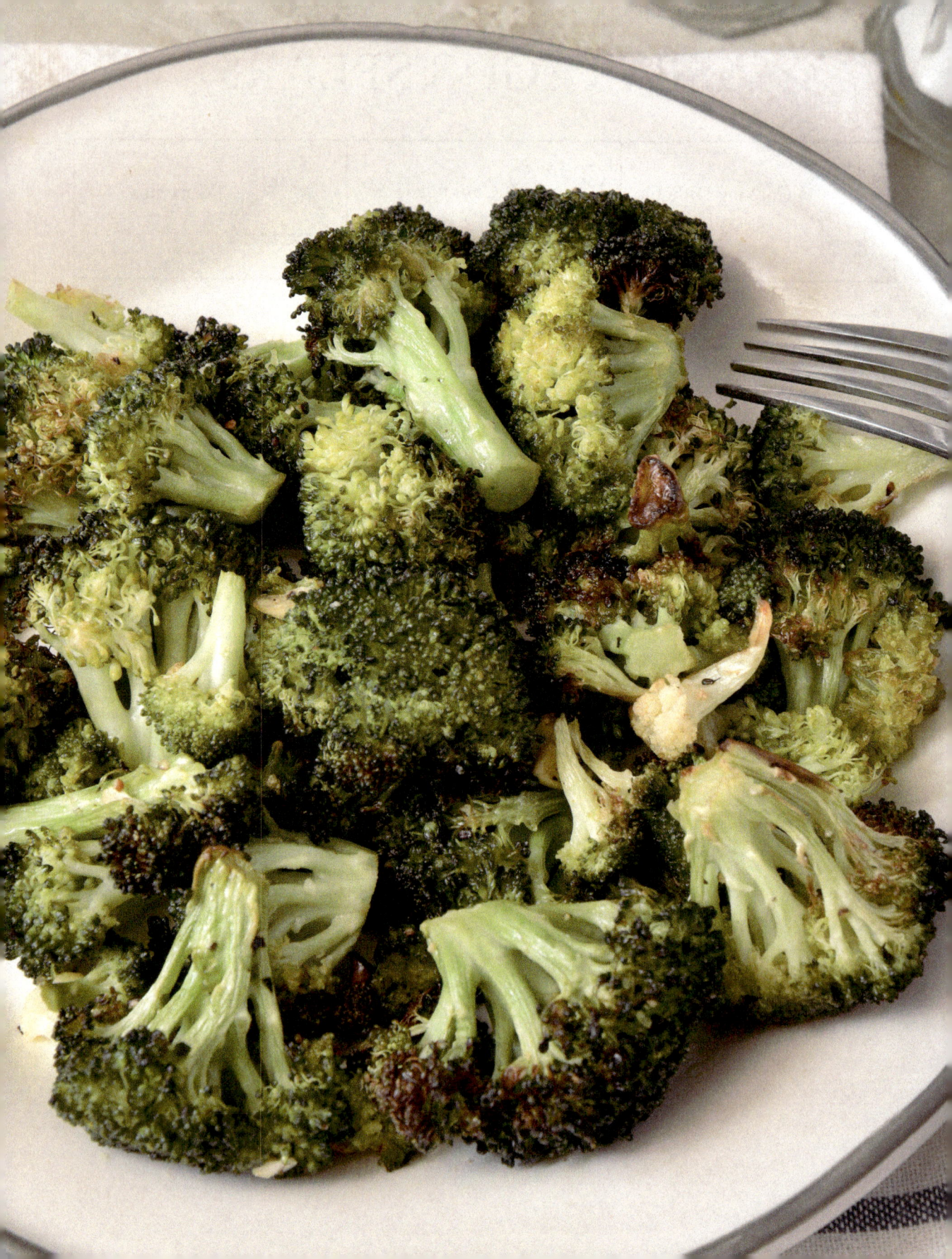

ROASTED BROCCOLI FLORETS

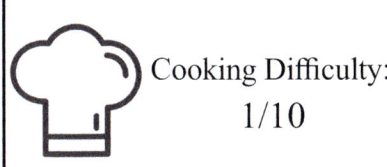 Cooking Difficulty: 1/10
 Cooking Time: 25 minutes
 Servings: 2

INGREDIENTS

- 2 cups broccoli florets
- 1 tablespoon olive oil
- 1/2 teaspoon salt
- 1/4 teaspoon black pepper
- 1/4 teaspoon paprika
- 1/4 teaspoon garlic powder
- pinch of red pepper flakes (optional)

DESCRIPTION

STEP 1
Preheat oven to 400 degrees F (200 degrees C). Line a baking sheet with parchment paper.

STEP 2
In a large bowl, toss broccoli florets with olive oil, salt, pepper, paprika, garlic powder, and red pepper flakes (optional). Arrange broccoli florets in a single layer on the prepared baking sheet.

STEP 3
Roast for 15-20 minutes, or until golden brown and tender.

NUTRITIONAL INFORMATION

Calories: 100, Fat: 5g, Carbs: 10g, Protein: 3g

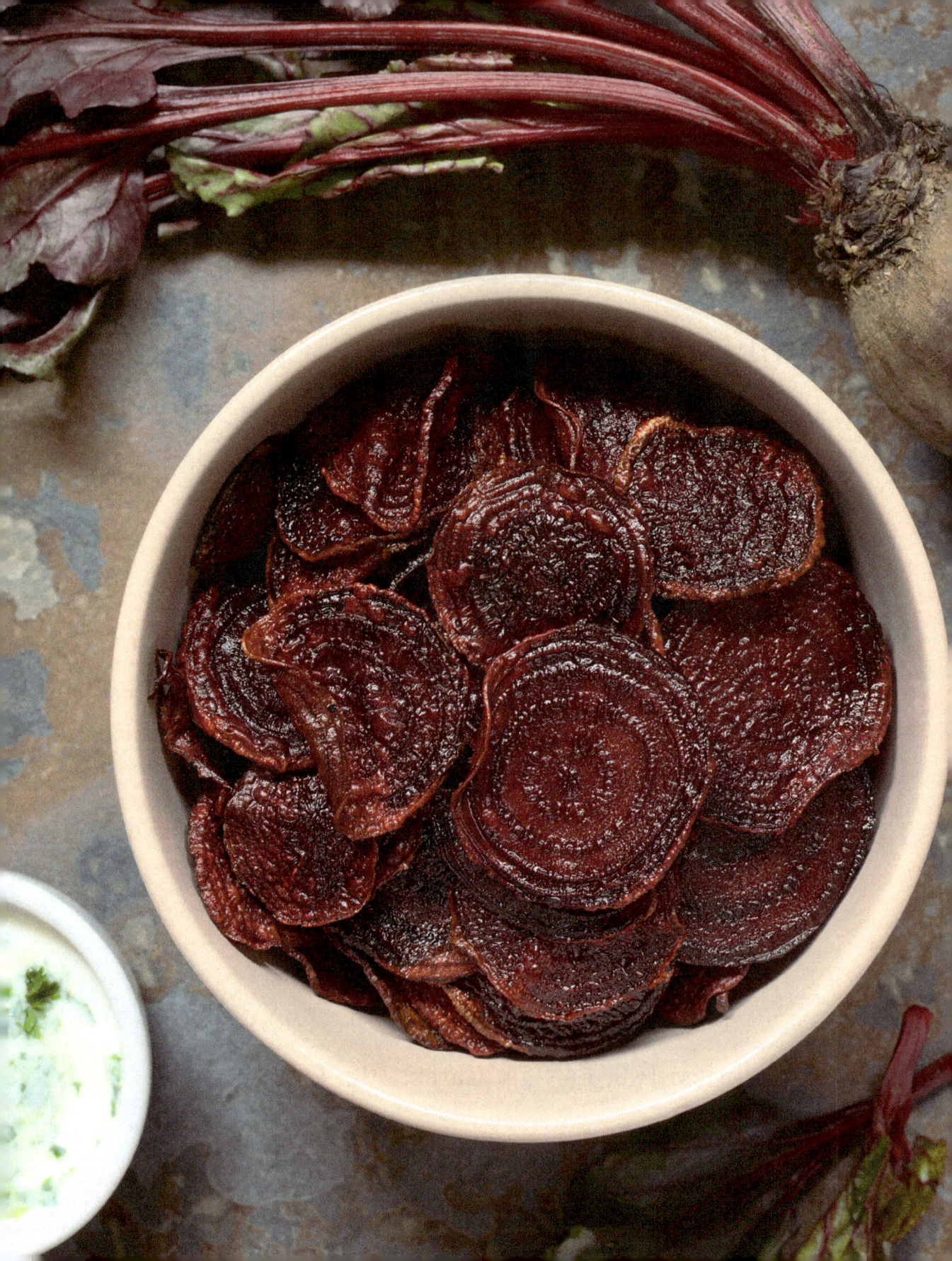

BEETROOT CHIPS

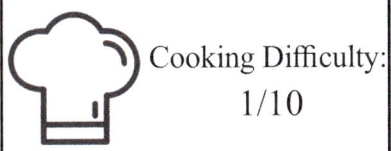 Cooking Difficulty: 1/10

 Cooking Time: 30 minutes

 Servings: 4

INGREDIENTS

- 2 large beets (about 1 pound)
- 2 tablespoons olive oil
- 1 teaspoon salt
- 1/2 teaspoon black pepper
- 1/4 teaspoon paprika (optional)

DESCRIPTION

STEP 1
Preheat oven to 350 degrees F (180 degrees C). Wash and peel the beets thoroughly. Use a mandoline or vegetable slicer to thinly slice the beets.

STEP 2
In a large bowl, toss the beet slices with olive oil, salt, pepper, and paprika (optional). Arrange the beet slices in a single layer on a baking sheet lined with parchment paper.

STEP 3
Bake for 20-25 minutes, flipping the chips once halfway through, until they are crispy.

NUTRITIONAL INFORMATION

Calories: 150, Fat: 10g, Carbs: 15g, Protein: 3g

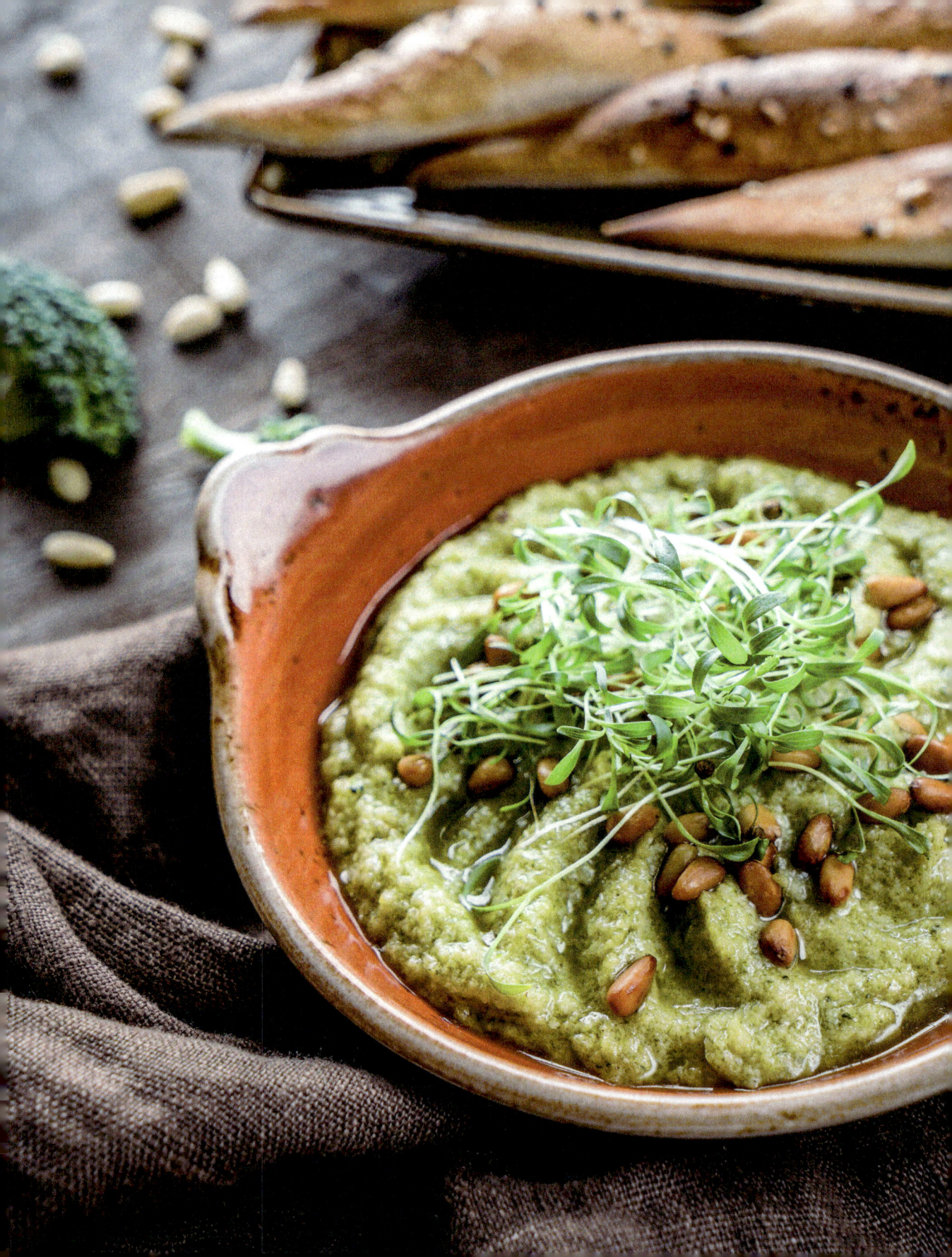

BROCCOLI HUMMUS

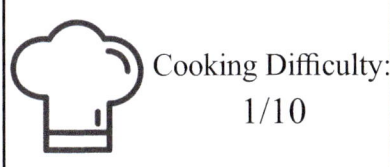 Cooking Difficulty: 1/10  Cooking Time: 8 minutes  Servings: 2

INGREDIENTS

- cup broccoli florets
- ½ cup canned chickpeas (or ½ cup cooked chickpeas)
- 2 tablespoons tahini
- 1 tablespoon olive oil
- 1 clove garlic
- juice of ½ lemon
- salt and pepper to taste
- 1 tablespoon water (optional)
- garnish: olive oil, paprika, parsley

DESCRIPTION

STEP 1
Bring a pot of salted water to a boil. Add the broccoli florets and cook for 2-3 minutes, until tender.

STEP 2
In a blender or food processor, combine the broccoli, chickpeas, tahini, olive oil, garlic, lemon juice, salt, and pepper. Blend until smooth.

STEP 3
If needed, add 1 tablespoon of water to make the hummus thinner. Transfer the hummus to a bowl and garnish with olive oil, paprika, and parsley.

NUTRITIONAL INFORMATION

Calories: 250, Fat: 15g, Carbs: 5g, Protein: 10g

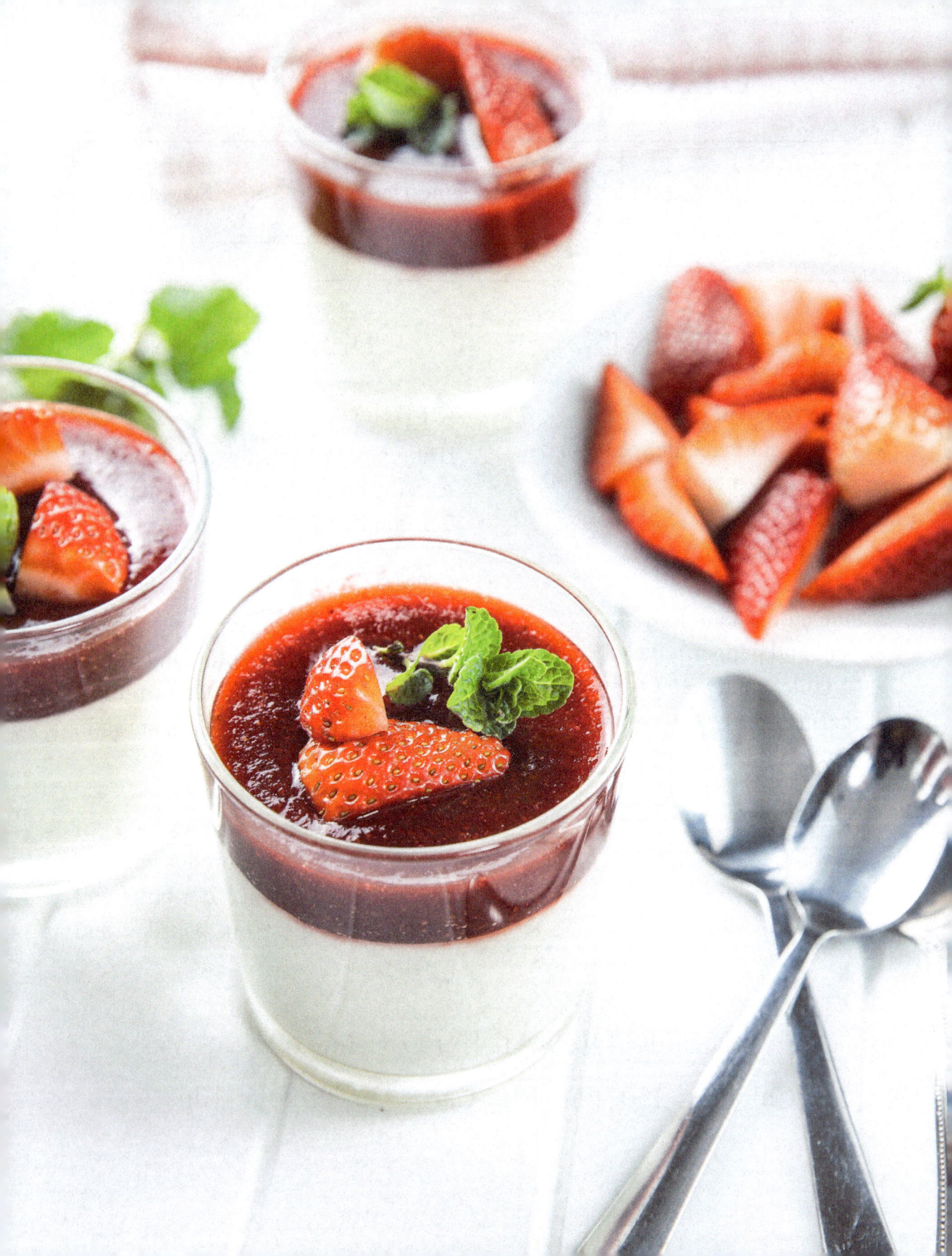

PANNA COTTA WITH STRAWBERRY COMPOTE

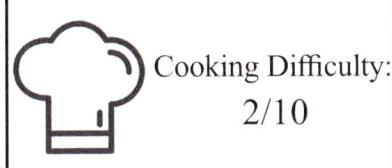 Cooking Difficulty: 2/10

 Cooking Time: 10 minutes

 Servings: 2

INGREDIENTS

for the panna cotta:
- 2 cups canned coconut milk
- 1/2 cup vegan yogurt
- 1/4 cup maple syrup, or to taste
- 1 teaspoon vanilla extract
- 1/2 teaspoon agar-agar powder
- 1/4 teaspoon salt

for the strawberry compote:
- 2 cups fresh strawberries
- 1/4 cup maple syrup, or to taste
- 1 tablespoon lemon juice

DESCRIPTION

STEP 1
Combine coconut milk, yogurt, maple syrup, vanilla extract, agar-agar, and salt in a saucepan over medium heat. Bring to a boil, whisking constantly, until agar-agar dissolves. Remove from heat and let cool slightly. Pour into 4 small ramekins or glasses. Refrigerate for at least 4 hours, or until set.

STEP 2
Combine strawberries, maple syrup, and lemon juice in a blender. Blend until smooth. Refrigerate for 30 minutes to chill. Top each panna cotta with strawberry compote.

NUTRITIONAL INFORMATION

Calories: 180, Fat: 8g, Carbs: 10g, Protein: 5g

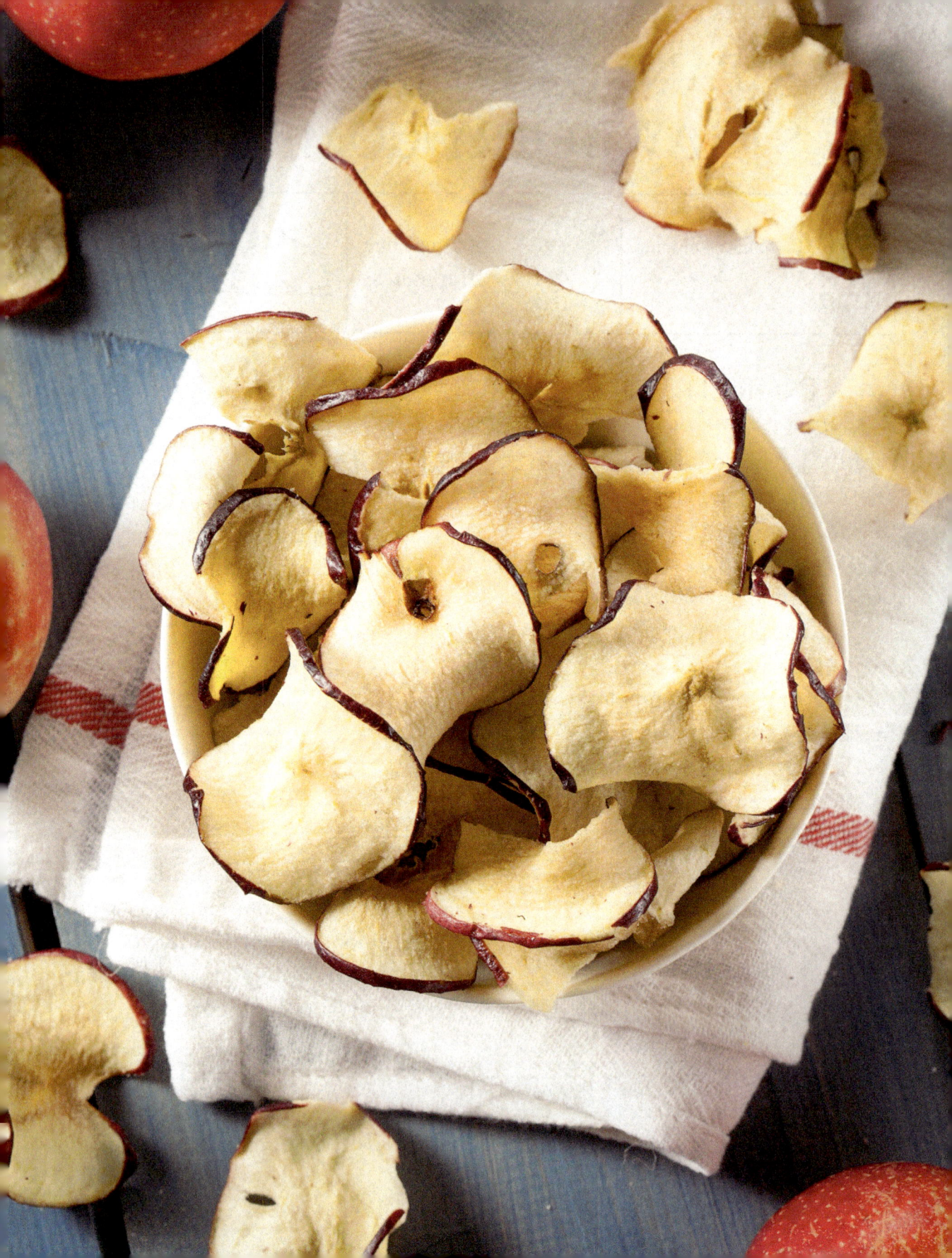

APPLE CHIPS

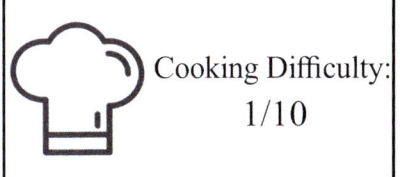 Cooking Difficulty: 1/10

 Cooking Time: 120 minutes

 Servings: 2

INGREDIENTS

- 2 large apples (sweet varieties)
- 1 tablespoon lemon juice (optional)
- 1/2 teaspoon cinnamon (optional)
- 1/4 teaspoon nutmeg (optional)

DESCRIPTION

STEP 1
Slice apples thinly. Drizzle with lemon juice (optional).

STEP 2
Add spices (cinnamon, nutmeg - to taste).

STEP 3
Arrange in a single layer on a parchment-lined baking sheet.

STEP 4
Bake at 200°F (100°C) for 1-2 hours until crispy. Cool and enjoy!

NUTRITIONAL INFORMATION

Calories: 150, Fat: 3g, Carbs: 10g, Protein: 1g

STRAWBERRY SMOOTHIE

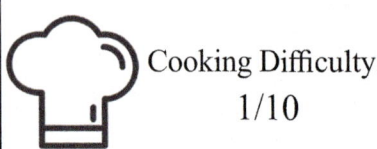 Cooking Difficulty: 1/10

 Cooking Time: 2 minutes

 Servings: 1

INGREDIENTS

- 1 cup frozen strawberries
- 1 banana
- 1 cup plant-based milk (such as almond milk, coconut milk, or oat milk)
- 1 tablespoon almond butter (optional)

DESCRIPTION

STEP 1
Combine all ingredients in a blender and blend until smooth.

STEP 2
Enjoy! You can drink the smoothie immediately or chill it in the refrigerator before drinking.

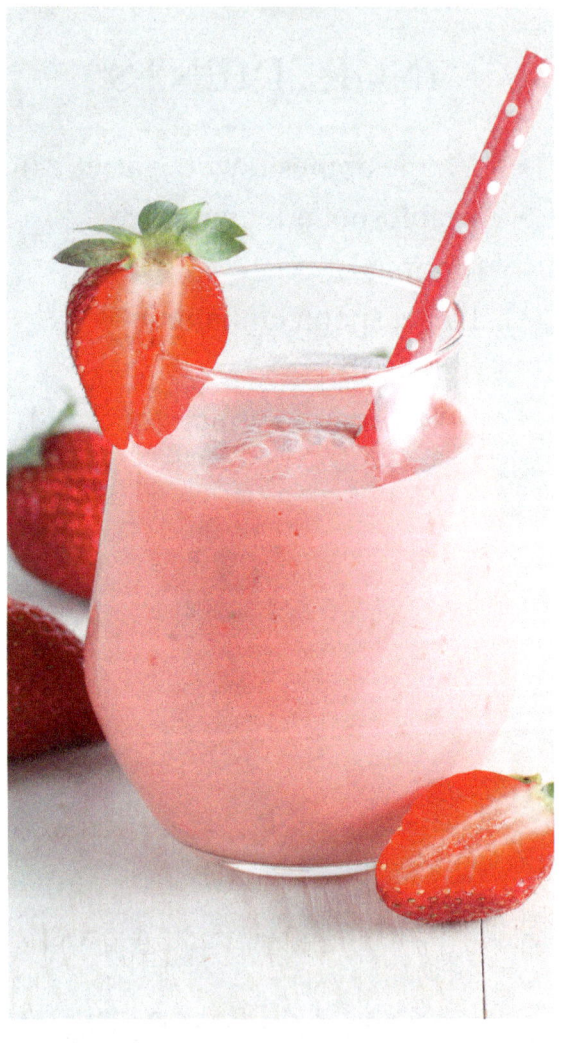

NUTRITIONAL INFORMATION

Calories: 350, Fat: 15g, Carbs: 35g, Protein: 5g

BERRY SMOOTHIE

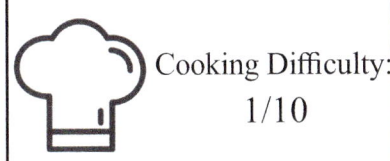 Cooking Difficulty: 1/10

 Cooking Time: 2 minutes

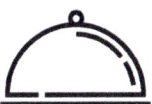 Servings: 2

INGREDIENTS

- 1 frozen banana
- ½ cup rolled oats
- ½ cup frozen berries (strawberries, raspberries, blueberries; your choice)
- 1 cup plant-based milk (almond, oat, soy)
- ½ cup water

DESCRIPTION

STEP 1
Combine all ingredients in a blender and blend until smooth. Add more water or plant-based milk if needed to reach desired consistency.

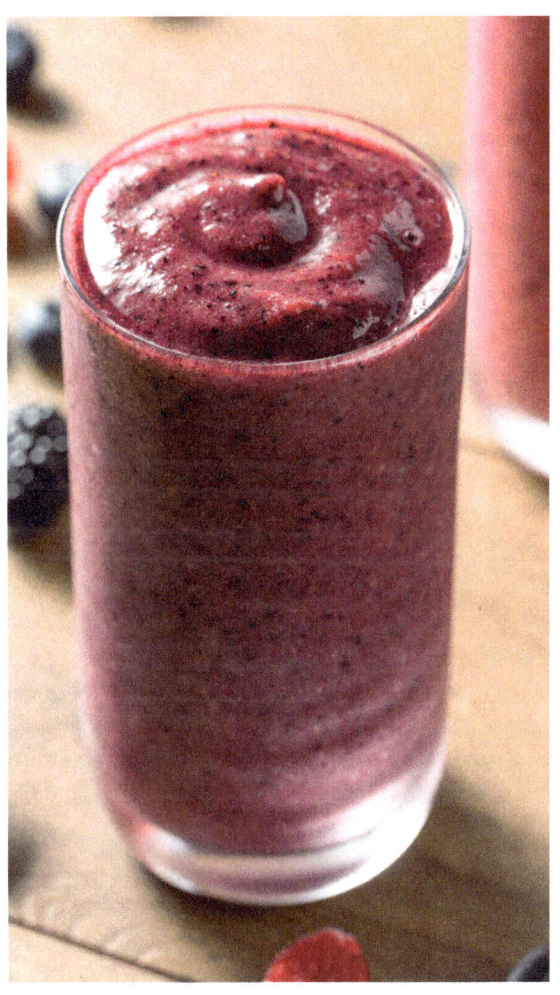

NUTRITIONAL INFORMATION

Calories: 300, Fat: 15g, Carbs: 40g, Protein: 10g

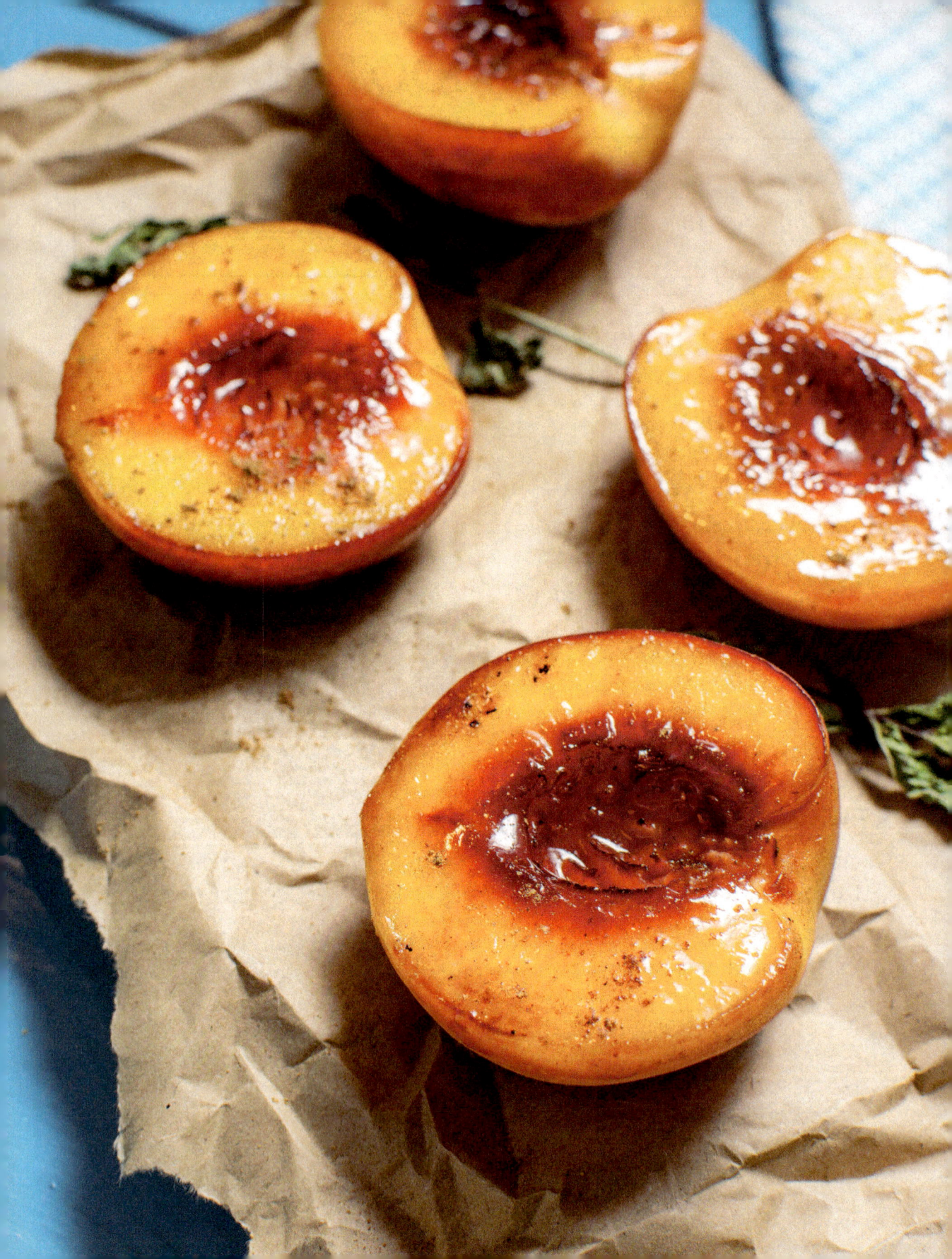

CINNAMON PEACH SLICES

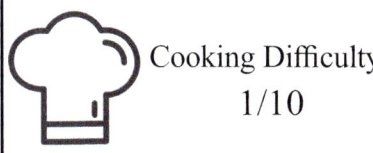 Cooking Difficulty: 1/10

 Cooking Time: 30 minutes

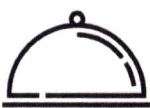 Servings: 2

INGREDIENTS

- 2 peaches
- 1/2 teaspoon ground cinnamon
- 1/4 teaspoon salt
- 1 tablespoon honey (or to taste)

DESCRIPTION

STEP 1
Preheat oven to 400 degrees F (200 degrees C). Wash and slice peaches.

STEP 2
In a bowl, toss peaches with cinnamon, salt, and honey.

STEP 3
Arrange peaches on a baking sheet lined with parchment paper.

STEP 4
Bake for 20-25 minutes, or until peaches are tender and slightly browned.

NUTRITIONAL INFORMATION

Calories: 216, Fat: 8.2g, Carbs: 27g, Protein: 9g

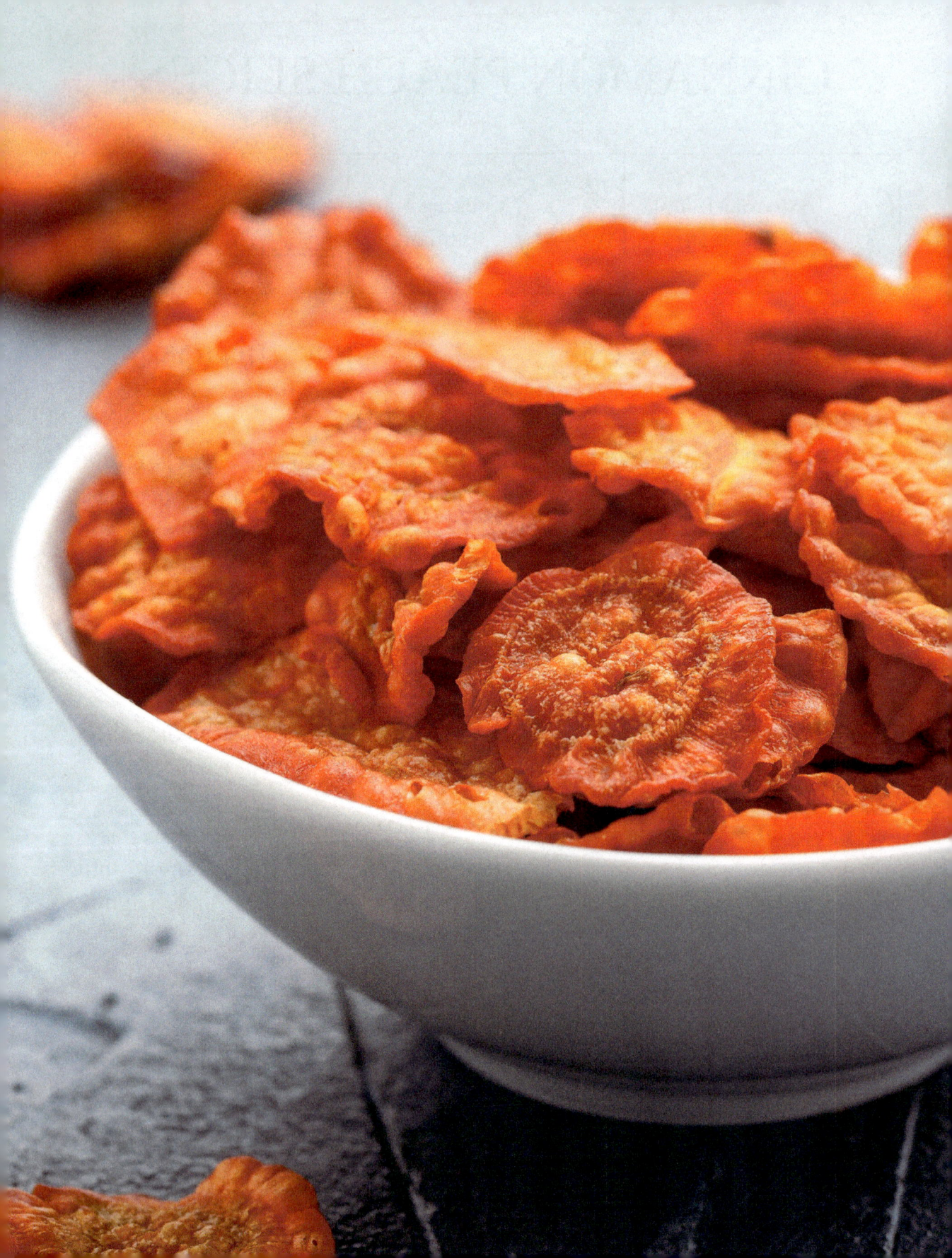

CARROT CHIPS

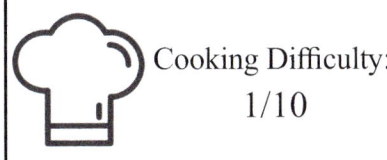 Cooking Difficulty: 1/10
 Cooking Time: 30 minutes
 Servings: 2

INGREDIENTS

- 2 large carrots
- 1 tablespoon olive oil
- 1/2 teaspoon salt
- 1/4 teaspoon paprika
- 1/4 teaspoon garlic powder
- 1/8 teaspoon black pepper

DESCRIPTION

STEP 1
Preheat oven to 350 degrees F. Line a baking sheet with parchment paper. Thinly slice the carrots. Use a sharp knife or mandoline to slice the carrots as thinly as possible. In a large bowl, toss the carrots with olive oil, salt, paprika, garlic powder, and black pepper.

STEP 2
Arrange the carrots in a single layer on the prepared baking sheet. Bake for 15-20 minutes, or until golden brown and crispy. Flip the chips halfway through baking to ensure even cooking.

NUTRITIONAL INFORMATION

Calories: 150, Fat: 5g, Carbs: 10g, Protein: 2g

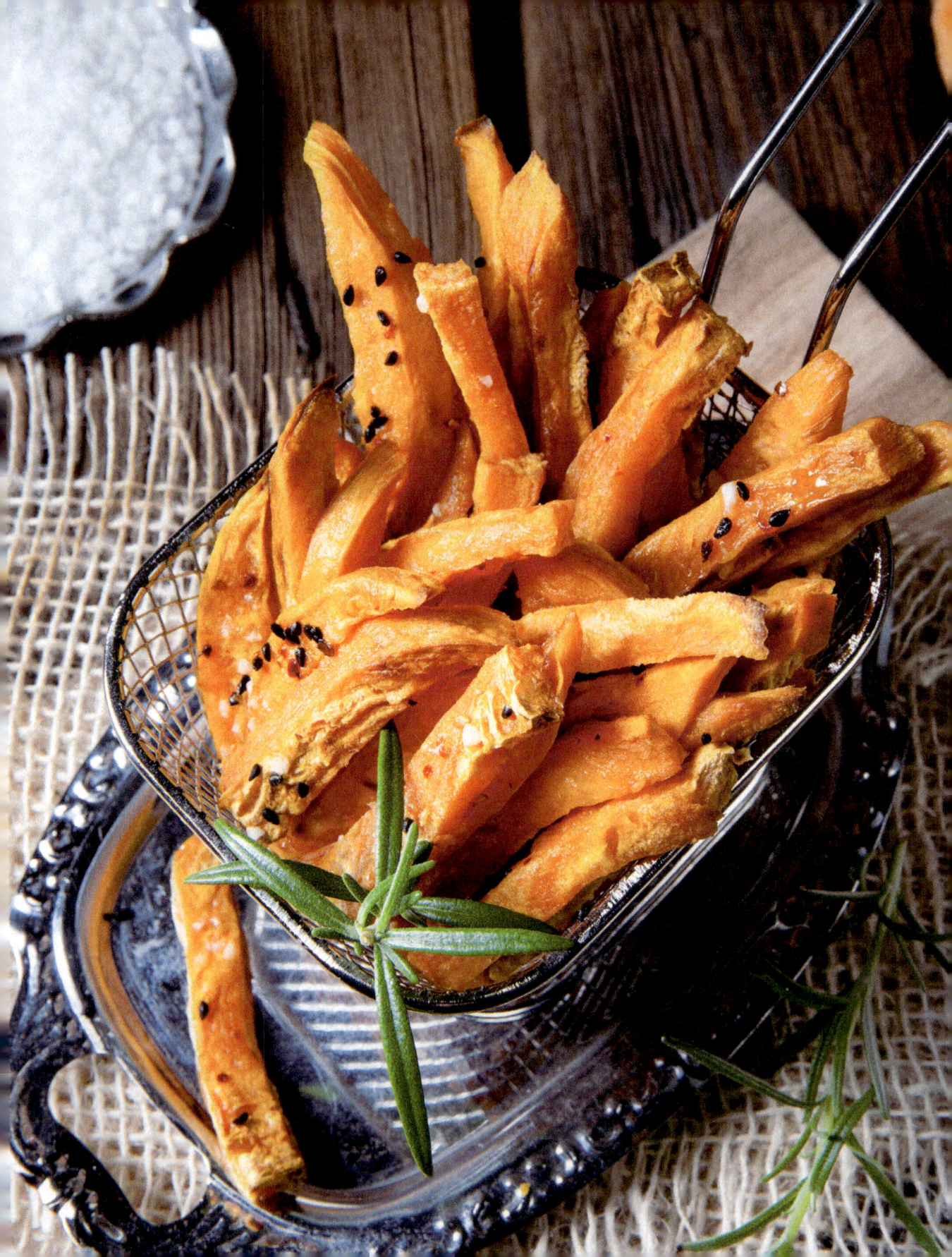

ROASTED SWEET POTATO

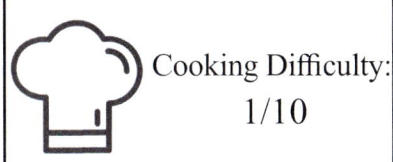 Cooking Difficulty: 1/10

 Cooking Time: 30 minutes

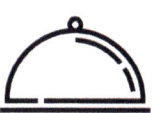 Servings: 2

INGREDIENTS

- 1 large sweet potato
- 1 tablespoon olive oil
- salt, to taste
- pepper, to taste
- 1/2 teaspoon paprika (optional)

DESCRIPTION

STEP 1
Preheat oven to 400 degrees F. Wash and scrub the sweet potato thoroughly. Use a sharp knife to cut the sweet potato crosswise into slices about 1/2-inch thick.

STEP 2
In a large bowl, toss the sweet potato slices with olive oil, salt, pepper, and paprika (optional). Arrange the sweet potato slices in a single layer on a baking sheet lined with parchment paper.

STEP 3
Roast for 20-25 minutes, flipping the slices once halfway through, until tender and golden brown.

NUTRITIONAL INFORMATION

Calories: 200, Fat: 8g, Carbs: 10g, Protein: 4g

CONCLUSION

As we age, prioritizing brain health becomes more vital than ever, and the MIND Diet offers a promising path to support cognitive function and overall well-being. Throughout this cookbook, we've explored not only the principles of the MIND Diet but also provided a wealth of delicious, nutrient-rich recipes designed to make healthy eating enjoyable and accessible.

By embracing the foods highlighted in this diet—such as leafy greens, berries, whole grains, and healthy fats—you can nourish your brain and reduce the risk of cognitive decline. The recipes included in this book are crafted with seniors in mind, focusing on flavors, ease of preparation, and nutritional benefits.

In addition to meal planning, we've emphasized the importance of adopting healthy lifestyle habits. From regular physical activity and mental engagement to fostering social connections, these practices work hand-in-hand with the MIND Diet to create a holistic approach to brain health.

Remember, every step you take towards healthier eating and living contributes to your cognitive vitality. Consult with your healthcare provider or a registered dietitian to tailor the MIND Diet to your individual needs, ensuring that you make choices that enhance both your brain health and quality of life.

By making the MIND Diet a central part of your daily routine, you empower yourself to embrace a vibrant and fulfilling life in your golden years. Let this cookbook inspire you to explore new flavors, enjoy nutritious meals, and prioritize your health—because your brain deserves the best care possible.

Samuel Hartwell

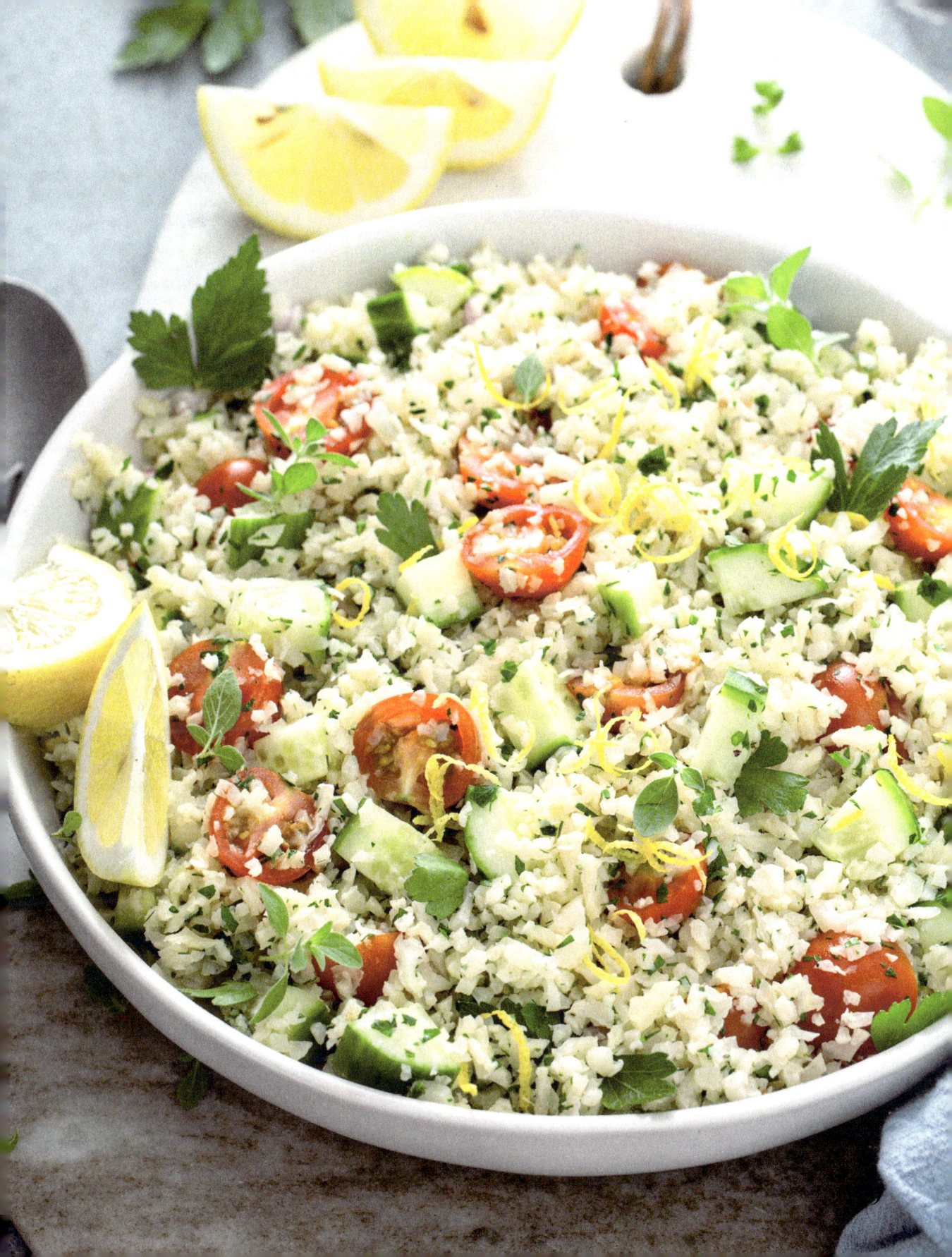

Printed in Great Britain
by Amazon